Dust, Scars and A Place to Land

Mindy M. Mather & Maranda Florer

Chapter One

Drake Rathburn splashed cool sink water onto his bristly face, the sharp chill biting into his skin and forcing him fully awake in a way sleep never quite managed anymore.

Droplets clung to his jaw and ran in uneven trails down his neck as he leaned forward, gripping the edges of the chipped porcelain sink. He kept his hands there for a moment, palms pressed flat, head bowed as he exhaled slowly through his nose.

The bathroom light flickered faintly overhead, humming with a tired buzz that matched the dull throb behind his eyes.

After a second, he lifted his head. His reflection stared back at him—tired green eyes dulled by years that felt heavier than they should have been. There were faint shadows beneath them, the kind that didn't go away no matter how much rest a man got…not that he got much.

His jaw tightened as he studied himself, like he was looking for something—something familiar, something steady—but finding only the same worn-out version he saw every morning.

His hand dragged over his bald head, slow and absent, before he let out a quiet sigh.

Five years.

Five years since he'd walked away from Dragonfly Academy. He'd been twenty-one then. Young enough to believe leaving meant escaping. Old enough to know better now because the truth was, he hadn't left anything behind.

The memories had teeth. They followed him. Lurked in the quiet moments. Slipped into his dreams—when he managed to sleep at all—and twisted them into something sharp and suffocating. Faces. Voices. The weight of it all. It never really let go.

Drake swallowed hard and pushed himself upright, turning away from the mirror like it had nothing left to offer him.

He preferred it that way—distance. From places. From people. From anything that might stick.

Being alone was easier. Cleaner.

Except for the nights when silence got too loud and the restlessness crept under his skin like an itch he couldn't ignore. Then he'd find a bar, or a roadside diner, or wherever people didn't ask questions. A glance, a smirk, a mutual understanding—and he'd end up in a place like this.

The Lone Ridge Motel.

He pushed the bathroom door open and stepped out barefoot, the rough carpet scraping lightly against the soles of his feet. The room smelled faintly of cheap perfume, sweat, and stale air—nothing unfamiliar.

Two women lay tangled in the bedsheets, limbs loosely draped over each other, their breathing slow and even.

One had an arm thrown across the other's waist, hair spilling across the pillow in a messy halo. They looked peaceful. Undisturbed.

Drake paused for a moment, watching them. A faint frown tugged at his lips.

He envied that.

Not them, exactly—but the ease of it. The way they slept like the world hadn't taken something out of them. Like rest came naturally instead of being something you fought for and lost.

He couldn't remember the last time he'd slept like that. If he ever had. His jaw tightened again, and he shook his head, brushing the thought away before it could settle.

It didn't matter. None of it did.

He crossed the room quietly, grabbing his ripped jeans from where they'd been tossed the night before. The denim was worn and familiar as he pulled them on, followed by the white tank top laying nearby. It hung loosely over his broad frame, the fabric stretched just enough to show the definition underneath without trying.

He moved with quick efficiency. He dropped into the chair in the corner, the wood creaking faintly under his weight as he reached for his boots. They were scuffed, broken in, molded to him after miles of road and dust. He pulled them on one at a time, tightening the laces with firm, deliberate tugs.

Routine. Something solid in a life that wasn't. Once they were on, he reached for his wallet, flipping it open and pulling out a wad of cash. He didn't count it—didn't need to. It was more than enough.

He set it on the side table near the bed. Payment for the room and enough extra for the women to get a decent meal when they woke up.

It wasn't guilt. It was just how he did things. No mess. No complications.

Drake grabbed his beaten-up backpack from the floor, slinging it over his shoulder.

It was worn, like everything else he owned, but it held what he needed—and that was enough. He gave the room one last glance.

No attachment. No reason to stay. Then he turned and slipped out the door, closing it quietly behind him.

Outside, the world was just beginning to wake. The sky was painted in soft streaks of early morning light, the sun barely cresting the horizon.

The air was cool, crisp, carrying that fleeting stillness that only existed before the day fully took hold.

Drake inhaled deeply, letting it fill his lungs. Then he exhaled slowly, watching his breath disappear into the quiet.

His motorcycle sat a few spaces down, dark and solid against the fading night. A Harley Davidson—his most expensive possession, and the only thing he allowed himself to care about.

It had been with him for years. Through every mile. Every town. Every restless night. Reliable and constant unlike everything else. He walked over, running a hand along the handlebar before swinging his leg over the seat in one smooth motion. The leather was cool beneath him as he settled in, securing his backpack behind him with practiced ease.

For a moment, he just sat there with his thoughts. Then he turned the key and the engine roared to life beneath him, loud and familiar, vibrating through his bones in a way that grounded him better than anything else ever had.

Drake didn't look back at the motel. Didn't think about the road ahead, either. He just pulled out of the parking lot and onto the long, winding stretch of asphalt, letting the tires catch and carry him forward.

Maybe he'd pass through here again someday. Maybe he wouldn't. It didn't matter. The road stretched out endlessly in front of him so he rode and let it take him wherever it wanted.

Drake didn't know how far he'd gone.

He didn't keep track of miles anymore—hadn't for a long time. The road blurred together after a while, one stretch of asphalt bleeding into the next, marked only by fading lines, rusted signs, and the occasional forgotten town clinging to the edge of nowhere. Time moved the same way. Morning turned to afternoon, afternoon to night, and somewhere in between he just kept riding.

The wind pressed hard against his chest, tugging at his tank top, carrying the dry scent of desert and dust. His eyes stayed forward, focused but distant, like he was watching the road without really seeing it.

He only stopped when the bike told him to. The low fuel light had been blinking for a while before he finally rolled into a gas station that looked like it had been dropped in the middle of nothing and left there to bake under the sun.

A cracked asphalt lot stretched out around it, weeds pushing stubbornly through the edges. The building itself was small, with faded signage and windows dulled by years of grime.

Drake pulled up to one of the pumps and killed the engine. The sudden silence rang in his ears.

For a second, he just sat there, hands resting on the handlebars, the faint vibration of the bike fading beneath him. Then he swung his leg off and stood, rolling his shoulders once as if shaking off the stiffness from the ride.

The heat hit him immediately. It clung to his skin, thick and unmoving, carrying the faint smell of gasoline and sun-warmed rubber.

He popped the tank and started fueling up, his gaze drifting lazily across the empty lot. A pickup truck sat parked near the side of the building, and an old sedan idled near the far pump, but otherwise, the place was quiet.

Good. Once the tank was full, he replaced the nozzle and headed inside. A small bell above the door jingled as he stepped into the convenience store. The air inside was cooler, though not by much, and carried the mixed scents of stale coffee, fried food, and cheap cleaning supplies.

Fluorescent lights buzzed overhead. Drake moved through the aisles without much thought, grabbing whatever was quick and easy—packaged sandwiches, a bag of chips, a bottle of water. Nothing that required effort. Nothing that lasted long.

Just fuel for him, same as the bike. He brought everything up to the counter, reaching into his back pocket for his wallet as he waited. The cashier—a middle-aged man with tired eyes and a name tag that had long since faded—rang him up without much interest.

Drake flipped open his wallet and paused. There wasn't much left. A few hundred dollar bills and some loose change. Not enough to keep him moving for long. His jaw tightened slightly as he stared down at it, doing the quick mental math he'd gotten used to over the years.

Gas. Food. Maybe a week or two somewhere cheap. Then nothing.

He exhaled quietly through his nose and handed over what he had for the items, tucking the near-empty wallet back into his pocket afterward.

Same cycle. Different place.

He stepped aside, grabbing his food, but instead of heading straight for the door, his eyes drifted toward a small corkboard near the front of the store. It was cluttered with flyers and handwritten notices—local services, rooms for rent, odd jobs.

Work.

That's how this part always went. He'd stop somewhere like this, find a job no one else really wanted, keep his head down, make enough money to move on. A few weeks. Maybe a month if the pay was decent.

Then he'd be gone. Like he'd never been there. It worked. Mostly because he didn't let it become anything more.

People always tried, though. Coworkers making conversation. Someone inviting him out for a drink.

Women lingering a little too long, offering flirtatious smiles that meant more than they said out loud and sometimes he'd give in to that part of himself. The part that didn't want to be alone all the time and bed them, but it never went further than that.

Couldn't. He wasn't built for staying. Didn't want the weight of someone expecting him to. His gaze shifted back to the counter.

"Hey," he said, voice low but steady.

The cashier looked up.

"You guys hiring?"

The man blinked once, then nodded toward a small stack of papers off to the side.

"Actually, yeah. Need someone for overnight shifts. Graveyard. Not exactly a popular slot."

Drake reached for one of the applications, glancing it over briefly. Overnight. Fewer people. Less talking. Less chance of anyone trying to get close.

Perfect.

"I'll take it," he said simply.

The cashier gave a small shrug.

"Fill it out, bring it back. Owner'll look it over, but if you're willing to work nights, you've got a good shot."

Drake gave a short nod and folded the paper, slipping it into his backpack.

Decision made. Just like that.

He grabbed his food and stepped back outside, the heat wrapping around him again as the door shut behind him. The sky had shifted while he'd been inside, the sun climbing higher, burning away the last traces of morning cool.

He walked back to his bike but didn't get on right away.

Instead, he stood there for a moment, staring out at the empty stretch of road beyond the station. Another stop. Another place he'd pass through without leaving a mark.

He had just enough money left to get himself a cheap motel room—something small, forgettable. Enough food to get through a few nights.

Then he'd start working. Earn what he needed and when he had enough, he'd leave. Just like always.

Drake swung back onto the bike, securing his bag before starting the engine again. The familiar rumble settled something in his chest, grounding him in a way nothing else did.

He pulled out of the gas station without hesitation.

Not toward anything. Just forward because that's all he ever did.

Chapter Two

The nearest motel sat less than a mile from the gas station, which suited Drake just fine. A squat, aging structure with peeling paint and a flickering sign that buzzed faintly even in daylight.

Exactly the kind of place he preferred. Forgettable.

He'd parked out front, killed the engine, and handled things quickly. The front desk clerk—a wiry man with nicotine-stained fingers and a permanent squint—had looked him over the way people always did, sizing him up without asking questions.

Drake had gotten the room without trouble. Getting it cheaper, though—that had taken a little more.

"Place looks like it could use some work," Drake had said flatly, glancing at the cracked tiles behind the counter and the sagging ceiling panel above the hallway entrance.

The clerk had followed his gaze, then looked back at him, interest flickering.

"You handy?"

Drake shrugged. "Enough."

That had been all it took. A short negotiation later, Drake had secured a discounted rate in exchange for doing maintenance—fixing whatever broke, patching what needed patching. It wasn't glamorous, but it meant he could stretch what little money he had left.

Once the key was in his hand, he'd headed to his room, dropped his bag just inside the door, and taken a moment to look around. It wasn't much—bed, dresser, small table, bathroom barely bigger than a closet—but it would do.

It always did.

He'd sat on the edge of the bed long enough to fill out the application he'd grabbed from the gas station, his handwriting rough but legible. Name. Basic details. Nothing more than necessary.

By the time he finished, he already had the next step lined up.

Job first, money next, and then the road again but before any of that—he needed a smoke.

Drake stepped back outside, the door clicking shut behind him as he leaned against the wall beside his room door.

The cigarette hung loosely between his fingers, one he'd bummed off the clerk before heading up.

He didn't smoke often. Didn't make a habit of it but sometimes when his nerves got the better of him, when things felt too still, too settled, like the ground beneath him was trying to hold him in place—that's when he reached for one.

He lifted it to his lips and took a long drag, the smoke filling his lungs, harsh and soothing all at once. He held it there for a second before exhaling slowly, watching the thin gray stream curl and dissolve into the dry air.

His gaze drifted outward.

There wasn't much around. A couple of small shops across the road. A diner with a sun-faded sign. A liquor store tucked into the corner of a dusty lot. Nothing flashy. Nothing worth stopping for unless you had to.

Which meant people didn't stay long. Good. That's how he liked it. He took another drag, letting his shoulders relax just a fraction as the nicotine settled into his system.

This would be temporary. A few weeks. Maybe a month. Then gone. No ties. No complications. Just like always.

His eyes moved lazily across the row of motel doors and then stopped. Another motorcycle sat parked a few doors down. Drake's expression shifted almost instantly, the faint calm he'd found snapping tight into something sharper.

His gaze locked onto the bike, taking in every detail—the make, the modifications, the subtle custom work that most people wouldn't notice but he did.

Because he knew exactly who it belonged to. A slow, irritated breath left him as his jaw clenched.

"Of all the—"

He cut himself off, dragging one last time from the cigarette before flicking it to the ground. The ember sparked briefly before he crushed it under his boot with a sharp twist.

Then he moved. No hesitation. His stride was long and purposeful as he crossed the walkway, boots thudding heavily against the worn wood. He didn't slow when he reached the door.

He pounded on it. Hard. Once. Twice. Again—louder this time. The door swung open and there he was. Donovan Deceasare stood in the doorway, taking an instinctive step back at the force of Drake's presence.

His long black hair fell loose around his shoulders, streaked with silver that caught the light unnaturally. The red contacts he wore gave his gaze an eerie, almost inhuman edge—but it was the tattoo that drew attention first.

A dragon, inked in bold, intricate lines, stretched across his cheek and slithered down his neck, disappearing beneath his shirt.

It marked him. Just like everything else from that place did. Drake's lip curled slightly as he looked at him.

"What are you doing here, Don?" he asked, his voice low but edged with something unmistakably hostile.

Donovan didn't answer right away and Drake let out a short, humorless breath, shaking his head slightly.

"Of all the places I stop," he muttered, his gaze hardening, "I find you here."

Donovan stayed quiet, his expression guarded.

Drake's eyes narrowed.

"Coincidence?" he pressed.

A faint huff escaped Donovan as he leaned one shoulder against the doorframe, trying—and failing—to look unbothered.

“I was here first,” he said. “So if you’re implying I followed you...you’re wrong.”

Drake studied him for a second, weighing the words, searching for something underneath them. He didn’t find anything convincing.

“Been staying here long, then?” Drake asked.

“A while,” Donovan replied.

Too quick. Too vague. Drake’s mouth twitched, unimpressed.

“Yeah,” he said flatly. “Sure.”

His eyes sharpened again, voice dropping just enough to carry weight.

“I bet Helena’s waiting on your report too, huh? My whereabouts, where I’m headed, how I look these days—”

Donovan didn’t respond. Didn’t deny it but he didn't confirm it either Just stood there and that silence said more than anything else could have.

Drake’s jaw flexed as something darker flickered behind his eyes. The name alone—Helena—dragged up memories he’d spent five years trying to outrun.

The headmistress of Dragonfly Academy. The one woman he never wanted to see again. He let out a slow breath through his nose and shook his head, stepping back.

"If she shows up here, Don…" His voice was quiet now. Controlled. Dangerous. "I'll ring your scrawny neck."

The threat hung in the air, heavy and real. Donovan didn't move or even try to argue.

Drake held his gaze for one more second—long enough to make the message clear—before turning sharply on his heel.

He walked back to his room without another word, each step carrying the same tension that had coiled tight in his chest the second he'd spotted that bike.

So much for quiet, temporary peace. The past had a way of catching up and it looked like it just had.

The first few nights passed without much trouble.

Drake settled into the routine faster than most people probably could have, but then again—he'd never been much for sleeping. The overnight shift at the gas station fit into his life almost too easily, like it had been waiting for him all along.

The nights were quiet and long. Still in a way that would've driven most people up the wall but not him.

He stood behind the counter more often than not, arms loosely folded or braced against the surface, his eyes drifting between the door, the windows, and the aisles.

Every now and then, headlights would sweep across the glass, followed by the low crunch of tires on gravel as someone pulled in.

Truckers, travelers, and the occasional local. They came in tired, distracted, sometimes talkative.

Drake kept things simple. A nod. A few words if necessary. Enough to get them what they needed and send them on their way.

No conversation beyond that.

The rest of the time, he kept busy. Stocking shelves. Straightening rows of snacks and drinks that didn't stay straight for long. Returning misplaced items to where they belonged. Sweeping the floors, mopping when needed, wiping down counters that never stayed clean.

It kept his hands moving and his thoughts from wandering too far into places he didn't want to go. By the time the sky began to lighten and the morning shift rolled in, Drake was already shutting things down for his end.

A brief exchange with whoever relieved him—usually nothing more than a grunt or a short "morning"—and then he was out the door.

Back to the motel and his room. Sleep came in short, uneven stretches. Four hours if he was lucky. Five if exhaustion finally caught up to him hard enough to drag him under.

The afternoons were for the other half of the deal.

Maintenance.

The motel didn't ask for much—just the usual wear-and-tear issues that came with a place like this. Leaky faucets. Loose hinges. Flickering lights. The kind of problems most people ignored until they couldn't.

Drake handled them without complaint. There was something satisfying about working with his hands like that. Fixing something broken and seeing it hold together again.

It reminded him of before of his days Dragonfly Academy. Before everything twisted into something harder. His father had made sure he knew how to handle tools, how to fix things when they broke instead of waiting for someone else to do it. Drake hadn't thought much of it back then.

Now, he was grateful for it.

It was one of those afternoons—dry heat pressing down, the air humming faintly with distant traffic—that he saw them.
Drake was crouched near the outside one of the rooms, a toolbox open beside him as he worked on a stubborn hinge that refused to sit right.

The metal scraped faintly under his screwdriver as he adjusted it, his focus locked in. Then movement caught the edge of his vision.

He glanced up and froze.

Ambrosia.

There was no mistaking her. Even after all this time. She moved across the lot toward the rooms, arms full of grocery bags, her posture slightly strained under the weight. One hand clutched the plastic handles while the other held onto a small child beside her—a little girl, no older than four, keeping close as they walked.

For a second, Drake just stared. Another piece of the past, stepping right into the present like it had every right to be there.

He let out a quiet breath and pushed himself to his feet, setting his tools aside without a second thought.

By the time she reached the walkway, he was already moving toward her.

“I didn’t expect to see you here too, Ambrosia,” he said, his voice steady as he reached out and took a couple of the heavier bags from her arms.

She let him but the second his voice registered, she stiffened.

“Drake…I…uh…” she stammered, clearly caught off guard as she looked at him.

Up close, she looked the same—and not. There were lines of strain around her eyes that hadn’t been there before. Something quieter in her expression. Worn down, maybe.

Her hand fumbled briefly in her pocket before pulling out a room key. Drake’s eyes dropped to it and then narrowed slightly.

Donovan’s room.

“You’re here with Don?” he asked, his tone sharpening just a fraction. He glanced down at the little girl standing close to Ambrosia’s side.

The child was quiet. Watching.

Her black hair framed her face in soft strands, and for a moment, Drake took in the details automatically—the resemblance to Donovan in the coloring, the posture—but then her eyes lifted.

Green.

Drake's brow furrowed almost imperceptibly.

He'd never seen Donovan's real eye color—not once. The unholy red contacts were as much a part of him as the tattoo and Ambrosia's eyes were brown.

"This your daughter?" he asked, his voice quieter now, more measured.

"Yes," Ambrosia answered quickly, pulling his attention back to her.

She offered no more information. Drake held her gaze for a second, then gave a slight nod, accepting it—for now. She turned, unlocking the door and guiding the little girl inside.

Drake followed without being asked, setting the grocery bags down on the small kitchenette counter.

"Are you guys staying here long term," he asked, straightening up, "or just passing through?"

His eyes shifted between her and the space, taking everything in.

"Because it seems really unusual that you're all here where I just happened to stop."

There was a beat of silence that stretched just a little too long.

Drake's gaze hardened.

"Almost like you knew I was coming here."

Ambrosia shook her head quickly, her grip tightening slightly on the little girl's hand.

"I don't—I don't know," she said. "Donovan's been… restless. Keeps moving us around." Her voice faltered, uncertain. "I'm just along for the ride with—"

She stopped herself. Cut the sentence short before the girl's name could slip out.

Drake noticed but he didn't press it.

Instead, he exhaled slowly, running a hand over the back of his neck before letting it fall.

"Yeah, well," he said, his tone cooling again, "like I told him—he better not bring Helena around here." There was no room for misunderstanding in his voice. "Or he's going to regret it."

The weight of that statement settled heavily in the room.

The kind of threat that didn't need to be raised to be taken seriously. Drake stepped back toward the door, his expression closing off again, the brief flicker of something more complicated disappearing just as quickly as it had come.

“I’m only here long enough to make some money,” he added. “Then I’m gone.”

He didn’t wait for a response. He turned, stepped out into the dry afternoon air, and pulled the door shut behind him with a quiet click.

The heat hit him again, but it barely registered. His thoughts were running a mile a minute and he wasn't sure what to think about having Donovan, Ambrosia, and their little girl there.

He only hoped he'd be getting out of there sooner rather than later.

Chapter Three

Drake settled into the rhythm of the place the way he always did—quietly, without drawing attention, without letting it draw anything out of him in return.

Nights at the gas station blurred together. The hum of fluorescent lights. The faint buzz of the cooler units. The occasional chime of the door as someone wandered in, half-awake and looking for caffeine or something to keep them moving down the road.

The front desk clerk at the motel had warmed up to him quicker than Drake would've preferred. The man—his name turned out to be Larry—had a habit of talking while Drake worked. About the motel, about the area, about nothing in particular.

Drake didn't encourage it, but he didn't shut it down either. He let the words pass over him, answered when necessary, and kept his distance but Larry had started greeting him with something that almost resembled familiarity.

"Got another one for you, Drake," he'd say, sliding a key across the counter or pointing toward a room number.

Drake would just nod, grab his tools, and get to work. The paychecks from the gas station came regularly—small, but steady.

Drake didn't deposit them. He didn't trust banks or anything that required his name to be tied down to a system he couldn't walk away from. Instead, he cashed them and folded the money into thick stacks, tucking it deep into his backpack. It wasn't the safest way to hold onto it—he knew that—but it was the way he'd always done things.

Cash meant freedom. No trail. No ties. The only exception was the prepaid card he kept tucked in his wallet, used strictly for gas at the pumps when he didn't feel like going inside. It was practical. Disposable.

But no matter how steady the routine became his thoughts kept circling back to Donovan, Ambrosia, and their little girl. It lingered in the back of his mind, quiet but persistent, like something scratching just beneath the surface.

Drake leaned against the counter one night, arms braced as he stared out through the front windows of the gas station. The lot outside was empty for the moment, the distant highway barely visible beyond the dark stretch of land.

His jaw tightened slightly. It didn't sit right. None of it did. Running into Donovan once might've been coincidence. Twice? Maybe but staying in the same motel long enough to settle in. Long enough that he needed to have Ambrosia and their daughter with him?

That wasn't random and Donovan wasn't the type to just drift without reason. Drake knew that better than anyone. Which meant there was a reason and he didn't like not knowing what it was.

His fingers tapped once against the counter before going still again. He hadn't seen Donovan in five years.
Not once. Not on the road. Not in passing. Not even a hint of him.

Same with Ambrosia and now suddenly they were here together with a child. Drake's brow furrowed slightly as that thought settled again. He thought back to their days in the Academy.

The Academy.

Even thinking the word left a bitter taste in his mouth. Cold stone walls, stricter rules than any prison, and that constant sense of being watched—measured, shaped, molded into something he never asked to be. Drake had never fit there. Not really. While the others fell in line, learned their roles, played their parts like obedient little soldiers, he pushed back.

Constantly. Recklessly. He broke curfew, skipped drills and mouthed off when he shouldn't have. He took whatever scraps of freedom he could find and held onto them like they were oxygen.

Then there were the girls.

Butterflies, they called them. Pretty, delicate things meant to soften the edges of the Academy's brutality. Meant to distract, meant to reward, and meant to belong to them.

Drake ran a hand over the back of his neck, tension creeping into his shoulders as one face rose clearer than the rest.

Ambrosia.

She hadn't been like the others—not entirely. There had been something quieter about her, something deeper behind those eyes that made him pause, even when he didn't want to. But she'd still come to him willingly. No hesitation. No coercion.

She chose him. That had mattered more than he ever admitted. At the time, it made everything feel…simpler. Cleaner. Like he wasn't just another part of the machine, taking what was handed to him. Like, for once, something had been real.

His lips pressed into a thin line. But even back then, there had always been Donovan.

Drake's expression darkened at the thought.

Donovan had watched. Not in an obvious way—not enough to raise suspicion—but enough that Drake noticed. He always noticed. There had been something off about it. Something calculated because Donovan had always had a thing for Ambrosia.

That much had been obvious and yet he never made a move. Instead, he nudged her toward Drake. Subtle comments. Convenient absences. Creating space where there shouldn't have been any. At the time, Drake chalked it up to cowardice or maybe some twisted sense of self-sacrifice.

Now? Now it felt like something else entirely. Something deliberate. Drake let out a quiet, humorless breath, his gaze dropping to the ground for a moment as pieces started shifting into a pattern he didn't like.

The day he walked away from the Academy, he didn't hesitate. Didn't look back. Didn't say goodbye. He burned that entire chapter of his life to the ground in his mind and told himself it was over.

Done. Gone.

He had been so sure he'd succeeded. Years of keeping his head down, drifting from place to place, working jobs that didn't ask questions. No ties. No records. No reason for anyone from that life to find him.

He'd built something close to invisible or so he thought. Drake's eyes hardened, lifting again as the realization fully settled in his chest, heavy and undeniable. If Donovan was here now, if he had somehow found him after all this time then it wasn't coincidence. It wasn't chance. It meant—

"He never stopped," Drake said quietly, the words tasting like steel.

A slow, cold understanding spread through him, tightening every muscle. Donovan hadn't just reappeared. He'd been there all along. Watching. Tracking. Following. Since the day Drake walked out of the Academy and thought he'd finally slipped free.

Drake's hand curled into a fist at his side, nails biting into his palm as a mix of anger and something darker coiled in his gut.

All those years. All that distance and somehow, it hadn't been enough. His jaw set, eyes narrowing as he stared ahead, no longer seeing the present—only the past bleeding into it.

"Why?" he murmured, though he wasn't sure he wanted the answer. Because whatever game Donovan had been playing back then, it clearly hadn't ended when Drake left.

He exhaled slowly through his nose. Something was off. He could feel it. The way Donovan had answered him. The way

Ambrosia had hesitated. The way she'd stopped herself from saying the girl's name and Donovan's "restless" moving them around?

That didn't sound like him either. Not unless something—or someone—was pushing him.

Drake's gaze hardened slightly.

Helena. The name surfaced uninvited, dragging a familiar tension with it. If Donovan was still tied to her, if he was here because of her, then this wasn't just coincidence.

It was proximity and Drake didn't like being found. Didn't like being tracked.
Didn't like anything that threatened the distance he'd spent five years putting between himself and that place.

His jaw flexed again before he pushed himself upright, grabbing a rag and wiping down the already-clean counter just to keep his hands moving.

He wasn't going to press it. Not yet. That wasn't how he worked. Pushing meant attention. Attention meant involvement and involvement meant getting pulled into something he had no intention of staying for.

No.

He'd do what he always did. Keep his head down. Work, save, and leave. When the time came, he'd find a way to shake Donovan.

Drake tossed the rag aside and glanced once more out into the dark, empty stretch beyond the gas station.

For now, though, he stuck to the routine because it was the only thing keeping everything else from catching up.

Chapter Four

It was one of his rare nights off from the gas station.

Not that it made much difference to Drake.

His body had long since adjusted to restless nights and fractured sleep. Even without the hum of fluorescent lights and the steady rhythm of customers drifting in and out of the station, sleep wasn't going to find him anytime soon. It never did when he wanted it to.

So instead of staring at the cracked motel ceiling for hours, he'd thrown on his boots, grabbed his wallet, and headed for the nearest bar. The place sat just off the main road, tucked between a half-abandoned laundromat and a diner whose neon sign buzzed faintly in the dark. It wasn't much to look at from the outside—weathered brick, dim windows, a crooked sign hanging over the entrance—but it was alive in that low, steady way bars in passing-through towns often were.

People passing time, people avoiding home, and people too tired to care who was watching.

Drake liked places like that.

No expectations. No questions. He stepped inside and was met with the familiar scent of beer, old wood, cigarette smoke baked deep into the walls, and the faint edge of cheap perfume drifting through the crowd.

The lighting was low and amber, just enough to cast everything in soft shadow. The kind of place where no one looked too closely. Perfect. He took a stool near the far end of the bar and ordered whiskey. The bartender slid it over without much interest, and Drake gave a short nod before taking a slow sip.

He settled in easily enough, one elbow resting against the worn wood as his eyes drifted over the room.

People-watching. A couple laughing too loudly in a booth near the back. A man slouched over his drink three stools down, staring blankly into the mirror behind the bar. Two women at the pool table exchanging playful shoves between shots.

Normal people doing normal things.

Drake watched it all from a comfortable distance, letting the noise wash over him without really hearing any of it. He'd only planned to stay for a drink or two and then leave but that plan unraveled the second someone slid onto the stool beside him.

He didn't need to look to know who it was. Still, he kept his gaze forward, his expression unreadable as he lifted his glass again.

"Shouldn't you be with Donovan?" he asked flatly. "Where's your daughter?"

Beside him, Ambrosia shifted slightly.

"They're at the motel watching a movie," she said. Her voice was smooth, familiar in a way he didn't care to examine too closely. "He knows I'm out tonight."

That made Drake finally turn his head and for a moment, he forgot whatever response he'd been about to give.

Her dark brown hair rested softly against her shoulders, catching the low light in subtle waves. The purple dress she wore hugged her figure in ways that left very little to the imagination, its low-cut neckline drawing his eyes to her ample cleavage before he could stop himself.

He looked away almost immediately but not before noticing. Not before acknowledging that she looked very, very good. A slow exhale left him as he turned back toward his drink.

"What you mean is," he said, voice dry, "he knows you're out keeping an eye on me."

Ambrosia let out a quiet sigh.

"Drake, I can't speak for Don, but I'm not here to spy on you."

There was something softer in her tone than he remembered. Something tired.

"Donovan and I take turns having a break from Al—"
She caught herself, her voice faltering for half a beat. "From watching our daughter," she corrected smoothly. "Tonight's my turn to go out."

Drake's brow twitched slightly at the stumble, but he said nothing.

"I didn't intend to run into you," she added, her voice lowering. "But I'm not upset that I did."

Then her fingers brushed lightly against the back of his hand. The touch was warm and intentional.

Drake looked down at it but he didn't pull away.

His jaw tightened slightly. He should have. He knew he should have but Ambrosia had always known exactly what she was doing.

"And maybe," she said, her mouth curving into a knowing smile as his eyes lifted to hers, "we can have a little fun."

There was no mistaking the invitation in her expression. No mistaking the memory it stirred. Drake's throat worked as he swallowed.

"Ambrosia, we can't," he said, though there was already less conviction in his voice than there should've been. "You're with Donovan, and—"

"That never stopped us before." The words cut him off cleanly. She leaned just a little closer, her perfume catching him—soft and expensive and familiar enough to stir memories he'd spent years burying. "And you know Don doesn't really care about that."

Drake couldn't help it. A crooked smirk tugged at one corner of his mouth because she was right.

Donovan had never cared. Not then. Probably not now.

Ambrosia smiled when she saw the reaction. Then she rose smoothly from the stool, adjusting her dress with practiced ease.

"I'm going to be in the ladies' room for a little bit," she said.

The way she said it made the meaning unmistakable. Her eyes held his for one lingering second before she turned and sauntered toward the back of the bar, hips swaying with unhurried confidence.

Drake watched her go. Watched until she disappeared through the restroom door. Then he sat there. His whiskey untouched now.

Every part of him knew better. This was a mistake. A complication. Exactly the kind of thing he spent his life avoiding. And yet the memory of her touch still lingered against his skin. The image of that purple dress burned sharp behind his eyes.

He exhaled hard through his nose and dragged a hand over his bald head, trying to shake off the urge coiling tighter in his chest. It didn't work. A few more seconds passed. Then Drake muttered under his breath,

"Fuck it."

The words barely left his mouth before he was already moving. He stood, dropped enough cash on the bar to cover the drink, and headed toward the back without another thought.

The low murmur of the bar faded behind him as he reached the restroom door and pushed it open. The heavy oak door of the restaurant's bathroom swung shut with a decisive thud, the sound echoing slightly in the small space. Drake's fingers fumbled with the ornate brass lock, his hands slightly unsteady from the wine they'd shared at dinner. With a satisfying click, the lock engaged, sealing them off from the bustling restaurant beyond. The moment he turned to face Ambrosia, the dim lighting of the bathroom cast shadows across her features, highlighting the hunger in her eyes and the slight parting of her full lips.

Before he could even register his next thought, she was upon him, pressing her body flush against his as her lips crashed against his. The kiss was immediate and desperate, a collision of pent-up desire that had been simmering between them all through dinner. Drake responded without hesitation, his mouth opening to hers as their tongues met in a frantic dance. His hands roamed the curve of her waist, tracing the delicate fabric of her purple dress that clung to her like a second skin. Her fingers tangled pressed into the sides of his head, pulling him closer as if she couldn't get enough of him.

The air grew thick with their ragged breathing and the soft sounds of their passionate embrace. Drake could feel his heart hammering against his ribs, each beat echoing the growing ache in his loins. Ambrosia's hands grew bolder, sliding down his chest until they found the cool metal of his belt buckle. Her fingers worked quickly, the buckle giving way with a soft clink that seemed to amplify the tension between them.

He was already hard and straining against the confines of his jeans, the fabric doing little to hide his arousal. Drake helped her free him from his jeans, his own hands joining hers in the urgent task. The moment he was released from the restrictive denim, he spun her around with a sudden movement that made her gasp. Her back pressed against the cold tile of the bathroom wall, the sudden chill a stark contrast to the heat radiating between them.

Drake's hands found the hem of her dress, hiking it up over her hips with deliberate slowness that made her tremble with anticipation. The fabric pooled around her waist, revealing the delicate lace of her panties. With one smooth motion, he yanked them down, the lace whispering against her skin as it fell to her ankles. He couldn't resist the temptation to admire the sight before him – the curve of her bare ass, the way she arched her back slightly in invitation.

A grin spread across his face as he raised his hand and brought it down in a sharp slap against her bare flesh. The sound echoed in the small bathroom, followed immediately by Ambrosia's yelp of surprise that quickly melted into a throaty moan of pleasure. The red imprint of his hand bloomed on her skin, a temporary mark of his possession.

"You're such a bad girl!" Drake exclaimed, his voice thick with desire. Before she could respond, he positioned himself at her entrance and thrust into her deeply, burying himself to the hilt in one smooth motion. Ambrosia cried out, her moan echoing off the tiled walls as he filled her completely. The sensation was overwhelming – the tight heat of her surrounding him, the way her body yielded to his, the desperate need that had been building between them finally finding release.

His hand came up to cover her mouth as he continued to thrust, pressing her fully against the bathroom wall. The tiles were cold against her skin, a stark contrast to the heat building between them. She moaned into his hand, the sound muffled but unmistakable as he kept up his relentless pace, their bodies slapping together with each powerful thrust. The bathroom filled with the sounds of their passion – the rhythmic slap of skin against skin, their ragged breathing, the soft whimpers that escaped her lips despite his hand covering her mouth.

Drake could feel her body responding to his, her muscles tensing and relaxing in waves as she neared her peak. He adjusted his angle slightly, hitting that spot inside her that made her cry out louder, her body arching against him. The pressure built between them, a coiling spring of pleasure that threatened to snap at any moment.

It didn't take long before Ambrosia pulled her face away from his hand, her head thrown back as she cried out in ecstasy. Her body shook with the force of her orgasm, waves of pleasure washing over her as she trembled uncontrollably. Drake could feel her inner walls clenching around him, milking him as she rode out the intensity of her release. Her legs grew weak, and he held her steady, his arms wrapped around her waist as she sagged against him, spent and satisfied.

As her tremors subsided, Drake felt his own release building, the pressure becoming unbearable. With a final thrust, he pulled out, letting his seed spill onto the floor at her feet in warm, sticky streams. For several seconds they stood there just breathing hard. The air was thick with the scent of their lovemaking, a heady mixture of sweat, perfume, and raw desire.

Drake knew that this was nothing more than a quickie, a stolen moment of passion in the midst of their busy lives. But as he held Ambrosia close, her body still trembling slightly from the intensity of her orgasm, he couldn't help but feel a deeper connection between them, something that went beyond mere physical attraction.

A sudden knock at the bathroom door startled them both, the sound sharp and insistent in the quiet aftermath of their encounter.

"Hurry up in there!! There's a line out here!!" A voice called out, muffled but clearly annoyed.

Reality came crashing back in, and they scrambled to compose themselves. Drake quickly tucked himself back into his jeans, his fingers fumbling with the button and zipper as he tried to regain some semblance of composure. Ambrosia pulled her panties up, the delicate lace now slightly askew, and smoothed her dress back down with a timid smile that didn't quite reach her eyes. She hurried into a stall, closing the door behind her so she wouldn't get caught as the one he was with.

Drake took a deep breath, running a hand through his disheveled hair before finally opening the door. He stepped out into the hallway, where a line of women stood waiting, their expressions ranging from annoyed to curious. A chorus of female gasps and giggles followed him as he passed them by without a word, his cheeks flushing slightly as he realized they must have heard everything. He made a quick exit, eager to escape before anyone could discover the mess he had made in the bathroom.

Chapter Five

Another week passed before Drake decided it was time to leave.

The decision came the same way it always did—not with some dramatic realization or restless burst of impulse, but with a quiet certainty that settled in his chest one morning when he woke in that stale motel room and knew he'd already stayed too long.

That was how it worked for him. There was always a point where a place started to feel too familiar. Too settled. The routine became too comfortable. The faces became too recognizable. People started nodding at him like they expected to see him tomorrow.

That was when he left.

Drake sat on the edge of the narrow motel bed, his backpack open in front of him as the first pale traces of dawn filtered through the gap in the curtains. He counted the cash slowly, thick fingers flipping through worn bills.

It wasn't as much as he'd wanted to walk away with. The gas station job had paid enough to keep him and he'd kept his spending minimal like he always did—cheap food, fuel, nothing unnecessary. Still, the stack sitting in his hands wasn't what he'd hoped for.

His jaw tightened. It would have to do. More importantly, he needed distance.

Distance from Donovan, Ambrosia, and from whatever strange, tangled mess they'd dragged into his orbit because the longer he stayed, the harder it became to ignore the truth gnawing at the back of his mind.

Plus after that night at the bar—after Ambrosia had pulled him into the women's restroom and reminded him exactly how dangerous old habits could be—Drake knew staying any longer was asking for trouble.

He'd made enough mistakes in his life and he wasn't interested in adding another. So he packed quickly. A few changes of clothes. Spare tools. The cash tucked deep into the inner pocket. Everything else arranged with the same careful efficiency he always used.

By the time he zipped the bag shut, the sky outside had shifted from black to dark gray. Perfect. Early enough to leave quietly. Drake slung the backpack over his shoulder, gave the room one last glance, and walked out without looking back.

The cool morning air hit his skin immediately. The motel lot was mostly empty, the world still half-asleep. A faint haze clung low to the horizon, and somewhere in the distance a truck groaned down the highway.

Drake crossed toward his Harley and set the bag down beside it, crouching to secure it to the back with practiced movements.

That was when he noticed him. Donovan stood a few spaces away near the door outside his room, one shoulder leaned lazily against the support post, a cigarette glowing faintly between his fingers. Watching.

Drake's irritation hit instantly. Of course he was there. He straightened slowly, exhaling through his nose as he tightened the final strap.

"Do you have a tracker on me or something?" he asked without turning fully toward him. Donovan took a long drag, the ember briefly flaring bright orange before he blew the smoke out in a slow stream.

Then he flicked the cigarette down and crushed it beneath his boot.

“I don’t need one, Drake.”

Drake turned then, his green eyes narrowing. Donovan shrugged lightly, his long black hair shifting over his shoulders. The silver streaks caught the weak morning light, and those damned red contacts gave him that same unnatural look Drake had always hated.

“I know you,” Donovan said. His voice was calm. “I know your habits. We spent years together at the academy. Got to know you pretty well when you weren’t beating me into the ground.”

He let out a dry, humorless chuckle. Drake didn’t smile. Didn’t even blink.

“Don’t give me that bullshit, Don.” His voice dropped low, sharp enough to cut. “I want to know how you’ve been tracking me since I left the academy.”

Donovan said nothing. Drake took a step closer and Donovan took a step back. Drake grinned knowing that he still intimidated him.

“What’s the point?” he pressed. “Dragging Ambrosia and your little girl all over the damn country following me when I don’t even know where I’m going?”

That was what bothered him most. Donovan following him was one thing, but Ambrosia? A child? That changed the stakes. It made no sense. Donovan only gave another slight shrug, like the question barely mattered.

"Better than staying in one place all the time."

Drake stared at him for a long moment and then something clicked. It was small. Subtle. A flicker in Donovan's expression. A tension around his mouth. Something that shifted behind those ridiculous red contacts just long enough for Drake to catch it.

Fear or maybe guilt. Either way, it was enough.

Drake's eyes sharpened.

"Are you working for Helena," he asked slowly, "or running from her?"

This time Donovan didn't answer right away and that silence told Drake everything. Something moved behind Donovan's eyes—too quick to fully read, but unmistakable. Drake felt frustration coil hard in his chest. So he'd been right. He just didn't know which version of right.

Was Donovan still Helena's obedient little pet, reporting back and keeping tabs like some loyal dog? Or was he running, dragging Ambrosia and their daughter from place to place because standing still made them easier to find?

Drake didn't know and Donovan clearly wasn't interested in clarifying. A harsh sigh left Drake as he scrubbed a hand over his face. He was done with this.

Done with questions that wouldn't get answered. Done with ghosts from Dragonfly Academy creeping back into his life.

"Just stay out of my way," he muttered. He swung his leg over the Harley in one smooth motion, settling into the seat.

Then he looked at Donovan one last time.

"And keep your woman away from me." The words landed hard. Donovan's expression tightened slightly, but Drake kept going.

"She's with you, not me." His jaw flexed. "I don't need you pushing her at me anymore."

The memory of the academy lingered sharp behind the words—Donovan's quiet encouragement, Ambrosia's knowing looks, all of it part of those twisted years Drake had spent trying to forget.

"I never did."

Silence followed. Heavy. Uncomfortable.

Then Drake turned the key. The Harley roared to life beneath him, the engine's familiar vibration grounding him instantly.

He didn’t wait for Donovan to respond. Didn’t care if he did. With one final glance toward the motel—toward the room where Ambrosia and that little girl still slept—Drake eased out of the lot and onto the road.

The tires caught asphalt. The wind hit his face and just like that, he was moving again. Leaving another place behind but as the motel disappeared in his mirrors and the open highway stretched endlessly ahead, Drake already knew the truth.

This wasn't the last he'd see of Donovan Deceasare.

Chapter Six

As usual, Drake didn't keep track of the miles.

He never looked at road signs long enough to care where they pointed. He didn't study maps or plan routes or pick destinations with any real intention behind them. He simply rode whichever direction felt right in the moment, letting instinct decide every turn.

That was how he'd spent the last five years. One road leading to another. One nameless town blurring into the next. No plan, no roots, and no reason to stop longer than necessary.

The steady growl of his Harley beneath him had become the closest thing he knew to peace. The vibration traveled through the frame and up into his body, grounding him in a way nothing else ever had. Wind pressed against his broad chest, carrying the scent of hot asphalt and distant rain somewhere he wasn't heading. The road was empty enough that he could let his thoughts drift. Not that he wanted them to.

His mind still kept circling back to Donovan. To the look in his eyes when Drake had asked about Helena. To the silence that had followed. That silence had said too much.

Drake couldn't shake the feeling that something bigger was moving beneath the surface, something he didn't understand yet and he hated not understanding things—especially when they traced back to Dragonfly Academy.

He gripped the handlebars tighter. The academy had already stolen enough years from him. It had no right to still be lingering in his life. He exhaled sharply through his nose and leaned into a curve, letting the motion of the ride burn away the frustration.

Hours passed that way.

The sun shifted overhead, slowly bending westward, and eventually the highway signs began pointing toward an exit. Without thinking much about it, he took it. The off-ramp curved gently downward, and as soon as the town came into view—

Drake froze. Not physically. His body stayed steady, his hands sure on the bars but something inside him locked tight.

He knew this place. Every inch of it. The realization hit all at once, sharp and strange enough to make his stomach twist. His eyes moved across the familiar stretch of road as he rolled farther into town.

The old hardware store still sat crookedly on the corner near the main light, its faded red awning sagging exactly the way it used to. The small grocery across the street looked untouched except for a newer sign. Even the cracked sidewalks looked the same.

Fourteen years and somehow nothing had changed. Drake slowed as he passed through the center of town, his green eyes narrowing slightly beneath the afternoon sun.

This was home or what had once been home. The town he hadn't seen since he was twelve years old. The place his parents had packed him up and sent him away from believing they were helping him.

His jaw tightened.

They'd thought Dragonfly Academy was some strict military school for troubled boys. A place that would straighten him out. Fix his temper. Beat the rebellion out of him and mold him into something respectable.

They'd never known the truth and Drake had never planned to tell them. Not then. Not now. The memories surfaced anyway. Being shoved into the backseat of his father's car while his mother cried quietly in the passenger seat.

The long drive. The gates. The towering brick buildings beyond them. The way his father had squeezed his shoulder and told him this was for his own good.

The way Drake had looked at both of them with enough fury in his chest to choke on it. Then they'd left him there and he'd hated them for it for years.

At first, they'd written letters. His mother's handwriting soft and careful, filling pages with updates about home and promises that this would all make sense someday. His father's notes shorter, practical, awkwardly affectionate in the only way he knew how.

Drake had ignored most of them. Sometimes he'd read them just to feel angrier. He almost never answered. Why would he? As far as he'd been concerned, they'd abandoned him.

Eventually, the letters stopped coming and Drake had told himself he didn't care. That he was glad.

That he never wanted to hear from them again. So why was his chest tightening now? He pulled into the parking lot of the small restaurant nearest the exit and killed the engine.

The sudden quiet rang in his ears. For several long minutes, he just sat there astride the bike, staring out through the windshield of his thoughts at a place he barely recognized and somehow knew perfectly.

Part of him waited. Listening for another motorcycle. For the familiar sound of Donovan's engine rolling into the lot behind him.

If Donovan was still following, this would be where he'd show himself. Drake wasn't even sure why he cared anymore. Whether Donovan was there or not didn't change anything.

His eyes drifted toward the far side of town, toward streets he hadn't walked in over a decade. Did his parents still live here? In the same house? Had they moved away after he stopped writing back?

Were they older now in ways he wouldn't recognize? Would they even know him if he stood in front of them? The thought made his stomach shift strangely.

He wasn't that kid anymore. That scrawny, furious twelve-year-old with waist-length red hair and too much fight in his bones.

That boy was gone.

The man sitting on this Harley was broad-shouldered and hardened by years of surviving things no child ever should have. His head was shaved smooth now. Tattoos climbed over his skin. His face was roughened by stubble and long roads and sleepless nights.

There was almost nothing left of the boy they'd sent away. Would they even see him in this version? Would they want to?

Drake swallowed hard. He didn't know why he cared. Maybe he didn't. Maybe this was just curiosity. A loose thread his mind had finally decided to tug.

Whatever it was, it had him reaching for the ignition again before he could talk himself out of it.

The Harley rumbled back to life beneath him. He sat there for one more second, staring down the road that would take him back to the neighborhood he'd grown up in. Then he eased the bike forward and went to find out what fourteen years had left behind.

The deeper Drake rode into the neighborhood, the tighter his chest became. It was subtle at first—a faint pressure behind his ribs, the kind that made it harder to pull in a full breath. But with every turn of the wheels, every house he passed that looked half-familiar and half-forgotten, the feeling sharpened until it sat heavy and suffocating in his lungs.

Anxiety. Real, sharp, unwelcome anxiety. Drake's fingers tightened around the handlebars. For a second, he nearly turned around. The thought hit him hard and sudden as he slowed at the next corner.

He could still leave. Could twist the throttle and disappear back to the highway before this became real. That was what he should do. What he always did. Run before anything could reach him but curiosity had already sunk its hooks too deep.

Fourteen years without seeing this place, without hearing from the people who had once been his whole world before they'd handed him over to Dragonfly Academy and driven away.

He needed to know. Not because he cared. At least that's what he told himself. Just because he needed answers. That was all.

He swallowed hard and turned down his old street. The motion sent a fresh wave of tension through him. Everything looked smaller than he remembered.

The sidewalks. The narrow stretch of lawns. The houses lined neatly side by side like they'd been arranged too carefully to ever change. Trees that had once seemed towering and endless now looked ordinary, their branches stretching over the road in lazy arches.

The whole street felt like a memory someone had shrunk down and left waiting for him. Drake's stomach twisted. He slowed further, his engine rumbling low beneath him as his green eyes searched ahead.

Then he saw it. The house. Exactly where it had always been. A simple two-story home with pale siding and dark shutters, tucked behind the same broad maple tree that had once dropped leaves Drake used to rake into giant piles every fall. The porch looked unchanged. The windows. The flower beds lining the front walk.

It was all still there. Only age had touched it. A little wear around the edges. Slight fading to the paint. Small imperfections time had left behind but it was still home or what had once been home.

Drake pulled to a stop two houses down, parking along the curb where the shade from a neighboring oak stretched over him and his bike.

Then he just sat there. Watching. His pulse hammered hard enough that he could feel it in his throat. Part of him expected nothing.

An empty house. Different people. A For Sale sign in the yard. Something to prove this place belonged entirely to the past. Instead, movement in the driveway caught his eye.

Drake's gaze sharpened instantly. There was a car parked there, one he didn't recognize. Newer than anything his parents had owned when he'd left. Different make. Different color.

For one disorienting second, he thought maybe strangers did live there after all. Then the man leaning under the raised hood shifted slightly and Drake knew him immediately.

His father. Older, of course. The years had settled into him in ways Drake could see even from this distance. Some gray threaded through his blond hair now, though it was still cut short and neat. His shoulders looked broader somehow, heavier with age rather than strength. There were deeper lines around his mouth, his posture carrying a faint stiffness Drake didn't remember but it was him.

Drake's breath caught. He hadn't prepared for how strange it would feel to see him alive and not frozen in some twelve-year-old memory.

His father was talking as he worked, his hands moving through familiar motions under the hood, explaining something and then Drake saw who he was explaining it to.

A boy stood beside him.

Teenage. Maybe thirteen, Fourteen at most. Tall for his age already, lanky in that awkward way boys got before they fully grew into themselves. His blond hair was lighter had been unmistakably inherited from their father, and he stood there watching with quiet focus while his father pointed at something near the engine block.

The resemblance hit immediately. Too immediate to deny. This wasn't some neighborhood kid. Not a cousin or a friend. No, Drake knew exactly what he was looking at.

His parents had another son.

His stomach dropped so hard it almost hurt. The boy nodded as his father said something, then reached forward awkwardly, trying whatever he'd just been shown. His father smiled faintly and corrected him, guiding his hands.

It was such a small moment. Ordinary and simple, but it hit Drake harder than anything else could have because he remembered that.

His father teaching him how to check oil levels in the driveway. Showing him which tools fit what. Patiently explaining engines while Drake half-listened and mostly just wanted to be anywhere else.

He'd hated those lessons back then. Now they felt like fragments of something stolen. His throat tightened painfully and then the anger came. It swelled so fast it nearly stole the breath from his lungs.

They replaced me.

The thought slammed into him with brutal clarity. They got rid of him. Sent him away because he was too difficult, too angry, too much trouble—and when he was gone, they started over.

A new son. A better one. One they could keep. Drake's fingers clenched so tightly around the handlebars his knuckles whitened.

The old fury he'd spent years burying roared back to life, hotter now because it carried something deeper underneath it. Pain. The kind he refused to name.

His jaw locked.

"Fuck…"

The curse slipped out under his breath, rough and bitter. His father and the boy hadn't noticed him. Neither had looked his way.

They had no idea he was there and Drake was grateful for that because if either of them looked over right now, If his father's face showed surprise or recognition or pity—Drake didn't know what he'd do.

He didn't want to find out. He'd gotten what he came for. Answers. The truth and it was worse than not knowing. With a sharp movement, Drake kicked the bike into gear and twisted it around.

The engine roared louder this time, shattering the stillness of the street. His father glanced up instinctively at the sound, too late to make anything out beyond a motorcycle already pulling away.

Drake didn't look back or slow down. He accelerated hard down the street, wind hitting his face like punishment as he tore away from the house, the neighborhood, the past.

His chest burned. His vision blurred for one dangerous second before he forced it clear. He had his answers now and they hurt more than fourteen years of wondering ever had.

Good. Pain was easier than hope. Drake leaned harder into the road ahead and let the town disappear behind him.

He was done here and this time—He wouldn't ever come back.

Chapter Seven

Drake ended up in a bar that night.

He hadn't meant to.

After tearing out of his old neighborhood, he'd spent the next hour riding aimlessly through the outskirts of town, the engine roaring beneath him while his thoughts tore themselves apart inside his skull.

He should've left. That had been the plan the second he'd twisted away from that street and left his father standing in the driveway with that boy—his replacement.

He should've gotten back on the highway and disappeared into the dark like he always did but he couldn't.

The anger was still boiling too hot beneath his skin, too tangled up with the hurt he refused to name. Every time he thought about his father leaning over that engine, calmly teaching another son the things he'd once taught Drake, his chest tightened until breathing felt like work and underneath the anger was something worse.

A quiet ache that had started the second he'd seen that boy standing there. He hated it. Hated that after fourteen years of telling himself he didn't care, one glance had proved how badly some part of him still did. So instead of leaving town, he'd ended up here.

The bar sat just off the main road near the edge of downtown, an old brick building with dim amber light spilling through dusty windows and a neon sign that buzzed faintly against the dark.

It looked older than he remembered. Then again, everything in this town did.

Drake had parked his Harley in the back lot where it sat mostly hidden beneath a dead streetlamp, then walked inside without really thinking about it.

Now he sat alone at the counter, broad shoulders hunched slightly over his drink, his expression locked into that cold, unreadable mask he wore so well.

The bar was half-full. Mostly locals. Middle-aged men hunched over beers after long shifts. A couple in a booth speaking quietly to each other. A group near the dartboard laughing too loudly at jokes that weren't particularly funny.

He sat near the far end of the counter where the light was dimmer, his large hand wrapped around a heavy glass filled with something dark and sharp enough to burn all the way down.

Whiskey.

The expensive kind by this place's standards, though Drake barely tasted the difference. He took another slow sip. The burn hit his throat, spread through his chest, and settled low in his stomach.

The bartender—a broad man with rolled-up sleeves and tired eyes—noticed when Drake finished his glass.
Without asking, he reached for the bottle.

Drake saw the motion out of the corner of his eye.
He could've stopped him. Could've waved him off and walked out right then, gotten on his bike, and left this town behind for good.

Instead, he said nothing. The amber liquid poured smoothly into the glass. The bartender set it down with a quiet nod and moved on. Drake stared at it for a moment before picking it up.

He hadn't intended to get drunk. That wasn't his style. Drinking enough to lose control had never appealed to him—not after Dragonfly Academy, where control was the only thing they couldn't fully beat out of him.

He just wanted enough to dull the edge. Enough to stop seeing that driveway every time he blinked. Enough to stop hearing the imagined version of his father's voice patiently teaching that boy things he should've still been teaching Drake.

He swallowed another mouthful. His jaw tightened. What had they told him? That thought had been gnawing at him ever since he'd left the neighborhood. What story had his parents given their new son?

Had they told him he had an older brother? Had they explained where Drake had gone or had they erased him entirely?

The possibility made something vicious twist in his chest. Maybe there were no pictures of him left in that house. Maybe his room had been painted over years ago, turned into that boy's room without a second thought.

Maybe his mother had packed away every trace of him and told herself it was for the best.

The glass creaked faintly in Drake's grip as his hand tightened around it. He forced himself to loosen his fingers before it shattered.

Across the bar, laughter erupted from a table near the jukebox. It grated against his nerves. He exhaled sharply through his nose and tipped back the rest of his drink.

The whiskey hit harder this time. Good. The bartender noticed and drifted over again.

"Another?"

Drake hesitated. Only for a second and then gave a short nod. The refill came quickly. He stared into it, watching the amber surface catch the low light. His reflection stared back in fractured pieces.

A bald head. Hard green eyes. The faint red stubble along his jawline.

Drake swallowed hard and took another drink before he could think too long about it. The warmth spread faster now, loosening the tension in his shoulders just enough to make him feel how exhausted he really was. Not physically. He could ride for another twelve hours if he needed to. No. This was deeper than that. A bone-deep exhaustion that came from carrying too much anger for too many years.

He'd spent all of those years blaming them. Hating them. Using that hatred to survive and now—now he didn't know what he felt. That uncertainty was worse than rage ever had been.

His eyes drifted toward the mirror behind the bar.
For half a second, he thought he saw movement near the door. A familiar shape. Tall and lean with long black hair.

Donovan.

Drake's whole body tensed instinctively but when he looked again, there was nothing there. Just another stranger stepping out into the night. Still, his pulse had quickened. The bastard could be here. Could've followed him all the way back to his hometown just like he'd followed him everywhere else.

The thought irritated him enough to make him drain half the glass in one swallow. He slammed it down harder than intended. The bartender glanced over but wisely said nothing.

Drake dragged a hand over his face, the stubble scraping rough against his palm. Enough. He'd had enough.

Enough drinks, enough memories, and enough of this town.

Tomorrow, he'd leave. Before sunrise and this time, he'd ride until this place was nothing but another blur in his mirrors.

That was the plan. It had to be because if he stayed—He might do something stupid.

Like drive back to that house, Knock on that door, and ask why they'd replaced him so easily. Drake stared down into what remained of his drink.

Then he lifted the glass and drank again, because for tonight, forgetting sounded a hell of a lot easier than knowing.

Drake should have left after that last drink. He knew it.

The thought had crossed his mind more than once as he sat there staring into the amber swirl at the bottom of his glass, letting the whiskey dull just enough of the hurt to make it bearable without quite numbing it away but he didn't move and the longer he sat there, the shorter his temper became.

The group by the jukebox had been loud all night, but now their laughter was starting to grate against his nerves like sandpaper dragged over exposed skin. There were four of them—local guys in their twenties, maybe a little younger than Drake, all of them flushed from beer and inflated by the kind of confidence that came from never having been hit hard enough to know better.

One of them kept slapping the side of the jukebox every time he picked a song, laughing too loudly at his own jokes. Another was butchering the words to some old rock song while the others shouted along badly enough to make the whole bar wince.

Normally, Drake would've ignored them.
Normally, they wouldn't have even registered beyond being background noise but tonight wasn't normal.

Tonight, every sound scraped at his nerves. Every burst of laughter felt pointed somehow, even though he knew it wasn't and when one of them shouted,

“C’mon, don’t be a pussy, pick something good this time,” followed by another round of barking laughter—

Something in Drake snapped.

The glass hit the counter with a hard thunk. The bartender looked over sharply, reading the tension immediately, but Drake was already moving. His stool scraped harshly against the floor as he stood. The room shifted slightly from the whiskey, but not enough to slow him down.

Conversations around the bar faltered as Drake crossed the room. He moved with purpose, broad shoulders cutting through the dim amber light like something carved from stone. The group near the jukebox noticed him too late. One of them turned halfway, his grin fading as he took in Drake’s size and the cold fury burning in his green eyes.

“What’s your problem, man?”

Drake stopped just short of him. Up close, he towered over the guy by a few inches, his expression unreadable in a way that made him instantly unsettling.

“My problem,” Drake said, his voice low and dangerous, “is that you haven’t shut the fuck up all night.”

The guy blinked. Then scoffed, trying to recover.

"Yeah? And?"

That was enough. Drake's fist connected with his jaw so hard the crack echoed over the music. The guy hit the floor instantly.

The room exploded into noise. His friends lunged at once. Drake met them head-on. The second guy swung wild and sloppy. Drake ducked under it and drove his shoulder into the man's ribs hard enough to send him crashing into a nearby table.

Wood splintered. Someone screamed.

The third caught Drake across the cheek with a lucky shot that barely turned his head before Drake answered with a brutal hook to the stomach followed by an uppercut that lifted the man off his feet.

He collapsed gasping. The fourth hesitated just long enough to realize he'd made a mistake. Then he swung anyway.

Drake caught his wrist mid-punch, twisted hard, and drove his elbow straight into the guy's face.

Blood sprayed. The bar had dissolved into chaos now—shouting, chairs scraping, people backing away fast enough to avoid getting caught in it and Drake barely heard any of it.

The anger had fully taken him now. Not because of these idiots. They were just convenient. Faceless stand-ins for years of rage with nowhere else to go.

Another man rushed him—one of the first guy's friends from somewhere behind—and Drake grabbed him by the shirt, slamming him into the wall hard enough to rattle the framed beer signs.

His fist drew back—And never landed. A hand clamped around his forearm like steel.

"Drake!"

The voice cut through the haze just enough to make him hesitate. Another grip caught his shoulder and yanked hard. Drake spun violently, instinct taking over.

Donovan.

For half a second, Drake didn't recognize him. Didn't process the long black hair streaked silver, the dragon tattoo winding down his face and neck, the red contacts glinting under the bar lights.

He just saw someone grabbing him and he reacted. His fist drove forward with everything he had behind it.

The punch landed clean across Donovan's mouth. The force snapped his head sideways. Donovan staggered back hard enough to slam into the doorframe as Drake ripped free and stumbled after him.

Donovan recovered fast, grabbing Drake around the middle and hauling him bodily through the back exit.

Cold night air hit them both as they crashed into the alley behind the bar. Drake shoved hard, throwing Donovan off him.

"What the fuck—" He barely got the words out before Donovan shoved him back just as hard.

"Calm the hell down!"

Drake swung again—Missed. His fist hit brick. Pain shot up his arm and just like that, the sharp sting broke through the whiskey and the rage like ice water dumped over his head.

He froze. Breathing hard. Chest heaving. His pulse thundered in his ears.

Donovan stood a few feet away, one hand pressed to his split lip, blood smeared across his knuckles. His red eyes—fake as always—watched Drake carefully. Neither of them moved.

The alley was suddenly very quiet except for Drake's ragged breathing and the muffled chaos still spilling from inside the bar. Then Drake looked at Donovan properly.

Saw the blood. Saw what he'd done and realization hit.

His shoulders dropped slightly. The fight drained out of him all at once, leaving only exhaustion behind.

"...Shit." The word came rough and low.

He dragged a hand over his face, wincing at the ache blooming in his knuckles. For a long moment, neither man spoke. Then Donovan spat blood onto the pavement and let out a humorless laugh.

“Still hit like a damn truck.”

That earned the faintest twitch of Drake’s mouth, though it wasn’t quite a smile. His breathing finally began to steady.

The haze was lifting now, the whiskey no longer enough to keep everything buried and with the anger fading, all that hurt from earlier came creeping back in to take its place.

Drake leaned back against the brick wall and closed his eyes. For once—He didn’t have the energy to run from it.

Chapter Eight

Drake didn't move.

He stayed exactly where he was, his broad back pressed against the rough brick wall of the alley, his chest rising and falling hard as he fought to steady his breathing. The whiskey still buzzed in his blood, though the sharp sting radiating through his hand was cutting through the haze fast.

His knuckles throbbed viciously. Every pulse of pain shot up his arm and settled deep in his wrist.

Good. The pain gave him something simple to focus on. Something cleaner than the mess still churning in his chest after seeing his father, after the bar fight, after realizing Donovan had once again managed to insert himself into Drake's life no matter how far Drake tried to run.

The alley smelled like wet concrete, old garbage, and cigarette smoke. Somewhere inside the bar, muffled shouting still carried through the walls, though it sounded distant now. Like it belonged to another world.

Drake kept his eyes closed for half a second more.

"Drake, I—"

The sound of Donovan's voice scraped across his nerves. Drake lifted his injured hand immediately, a low grunt slipping through his teeth at the motion.

"Go away, Donovan." His voice came out rough, flat, final.

For a second, he thought Donovan might actually listen but of course he didn't.

"No, Drake."

There was something firmer in Donovan's voice now. Something less cautious than before.

"I want you to stay away from my wife."

Drake's eyes cracked open. Slowly. He turned his head just enough to look at him.

Donovan stood a few feet away under the weak yellow spill of the alley light, one hand still pressed loosely against his split lip. Blood darkened the corner of his mouth and smeared across his chin, but he looked more irritated than hurt.

The sight should have been satisfying. Instead, it only annoyed Drake more.

"Ambrosia is my wife," Donovan continued, his jaw tightening. "You have no right to—"

"Ambrosia propositioned me." Drake cut him off cold. The words dropped heavy into the narrow space between them. Donovan went still. Drake pushed off the wall slightly, enough to stand straighter despite the pull of pain in his hand.

"I just gave her what she wanted," he said, his voice sharp now. His eyes locked onto Donovan's with open challenge. "She said you wouldn't care."

For a moment, Donovan said nothing. His expression shifted—something tightening behind those unnatural lenses. Then he exhaled sharply.

"Yeah, well…" His voice was quieter now, harder somehow. "I do."

Drake's eyes narrowed.

"And I made sure she understands that." The words hit like a slap. A sudden coldness flooded Drake's chest. "She won't come to you for that again."

Drake straightened fully. The exhaustion vanished. His entire body went taut.

"What did you do?" The question came low and dangerous.

Donovan's posture shifted immediately. Instinctive retreat.

"Drake—"

"Don't tell me you hurt her, Don." Drake's voice dropped lower still, the edge in it enough to make Donovan take a step back.

"You know I don't stand for that shit."

Donovan's hands lifted slightly, defensive.

"She crossed a line." The explanation came too quickly. Too rehearsed.

Drake's stomach turned.

"I just did what we were taught—"

He never finished. Drake moved so fast Donovan barely had time to register it. One second there was space between them—The next Drake's good hand had a fistful of Donovan's shirt, hauling him violently forward until his boots barely touched the pavement.

Donovan let out a startled gasp, forced onto his tiptoes as Drake lifted him higher. His face was inches from Donovan's now, eyes blazing. Every word that followed came quiet and deadly.

"You better not ever lay a hand on her like that again.

Donovan swallowed hard. Drake's grip tightened.

"Or you'll regret following me around."

The alley had gone deathly still. Even the distant noise from the bar seemed to disappear.

Drake leaned closer, his voice dropping to a near growl.

"I will know." The promise carried absolute certainty. "And whatever you do to her…" His jaw flexed. "I'll do to you ten times worse."

Donovan's breathing had gone shallow. His face had lost what little color it had. Drake held his gaze for another long second before asking, each word deliberate:

"Am I clear?"

Donovan's throat bobbed.

"Crystal."

Drake studied him. Making sure he meant it. Then he gave one short nod.

"Good." His eyes sharpened further. "Same goes for your little girl."

That hit Donovan visibly harder. Drake noticed and pressed.

"I better not ever see a mark on her." Then he released him so forcefully that Donovan stumbled backward several steps, nearly losing his footing before catching himself against the wall. He sucked in a rough breath, one hand clutching at his wrinkled shirt.

Drake turned immediately. Done with this. Done with him. He made it three steps toward the alley mouth before Donovan's voice stopped him.

"Your hand needs a doctor."

Drake paused. Didn't turn.

"It's probably broken."

Drake glanced down. His knuckles were already swelling badly, the skin split across two of them. His wrist looked wrong—just slightly off. Shit. Before he could dismiss it, Donovan added:

"And you're drunk."

That got a humorless snort from Drake.

"You shouldn't ride tonight."

Drake finally looked back over his shoulder. Donovan had straightened again, though he kept his distance this time.

The caution in his posture was obvious.

"Come with me," he said carefully. "We'll take you to the hospital in our van."

Drake stared at him. His first instinct was to refuse. Hell no.

The idea of climbing into a van with Donovan—possibly with Ambrosia there too—felt like a special kind of punishment but then his hand throbbed again, sharp enough to make his stomach twist and Donovan was right.

He was drunk enough that getting on his bike tonight would be stupid. Drake hated admitting that. He stood there for a long moment, weighing his options. The alley was quiet again.

The cool night air brushed against his overheated skin. Finally, he let out another low grunt.

"Fine."

The word sounded more like a threat than agreement. Donovan visibly relaxed, though only slightly.

Drake shot him one final warning look.

"This doesn't mean I like you."

To his credit, Donovan gave the faintest twitch of a humorless smile.

"Yeah," he muttered, rubbing his throat. "I got that."

Drake rolled his eyes and started walking and for the first time ever he followed Donovan somewhere.

The cast made everything harder.

Drake had left the hospital just before dawn with his right hand wrapped in thick white plaster from his knuckles down past his wrist, the rigid weight of it awkward and unfamiliar.

The doctor had been annoyingly cheerful when he'd confirmed what Drake had already suspected—a clean break across the hand from punching brick after missing Donovan's face in the alley.

Six weeks, maybe less if he didn't do anything stupid.

Drake had nearly laughed at that. Doing something stupid was practically a requirement for his existence. Still, the cast was there now, heavy and inconvenient, and it made gripping the throttle of his Harley a miserable exercise in adaptation.

He hated it.

Every twist of the handlebars sent a dull ache through his arm. Every shift of balance reminded him that his body wasn't working the way it was supposed to but Drake Rathburn had spent too many years forcing himself through worse pain to let something as simple as a broken hand stop him.

So the second the sun rose high enough to wash the streets of his hometown in pale gold, he was gone.

He didn't look back.

Not at the quiet neighborhood where his parents and their new son were probably waking up to another ordinary morning.

He didn't need another look at what fourteen years had turned his life into.

The Harley growled beneath him as he pulled onto the highway, the vibration climbing through the frame and into his body like an old friend reminding him how to breathe.

The road opened ahead. Endless and familiar. Exactly where he belonged. He kept riding. Mile after mile after mile. The pain in his hand faded into background noise, replaced by the rhythmic roar of the engine and the dry rush of wind against his face.

His only real plan was distance. He wanted as much of it as possible between himself and that town before he stopped.

Eventually, when his body finally forced him to admit he needed rest, he'd find some cheap roadside motel, hole up for a month, let the hand heal, save his cash, and disappear again once he was whole enough to ride properly.

Same routine. Same life. Simple and predictable and yet—He wasn't alone this time. Drake could hear Donovan's bike behind him whenever the highway quieted enough.

That low mechanical growl stayed close but never too close, hovering a few car lengths back like some patient shadow refusing to disappear and farther behind that, Ambrosia followed in their beat-up van, steady and careful behind the wheel.

He'd caught brief glimpses of it in his mirrors during gas stops—the faded blue paint, the windshield cluttered with old parking stickers, the little shape of their daughter visible through the backseat window in her booster seat. Buckled in. Quietly watching the world roll by. Drake still didn't know the girl's name.

The realization struck him harder than it should have.

He'd been around them for weeks now. Shared motel walls, conversations, warnings, fights, and one mistake with Ambrosia that he'd already shoved firmly into the category of things he would never think too hard about and somehow he still didn't know the kid's name.

That felt…strange. Wrong, somehow. He pushed the thought aside. It wasn't his business. None of this was.

He should have been irritated by their presence. Should have hated the fact that Donovan was still following him across state lines like some half-trained stray refusing to take a hint. Should have snapped at Ambrosia every time she pulled alongside at rest stops and asked if he needed anything.

Should have resented every mile they shared. Instead—He didn't and that annoyed him most of all. Because somewhere beneath all his resistance, there was something unexpectedly steady about having them there.

At the first gas stop just after noon, Drake had pulled off stiffly and dismounted with a muttered curse when his cast caught awkwardly against the bars.

Before he could even fully straighten, Ambrosia was there.

"Need help?" Her voice was light, casual. Like nothing complicated had ever happened between them. Drake glanced at her. She wore jeans and a fitted black tank top today, her dark hair tied loosely back against the heat.

There was no trace of bruising on her, but she winced some whenever she moved a certain direction. It angered Drake that Donovan would hurt her, but he didn't blame him entirely.

It was what they'd been taught and Drake knew that Donovan hadn't fully broken free from those teachings.

He shook his head.

“I’m fine.”

Ambrosia gave him a knowing look that said she didn’t believe him for a second but she let it go.

Their daughter was climbing carefully out of the van now, Donovan helping her down with quiet patience that Drake wouldn’t have expected from him once upon a time. The little girl looked up at Donovan and smiled.

Drake looked away before something uncomfortable settled too deeply in his chest. The thought felt too complicated to examine. So he fueled up, paid in cash one-handed, and got back on the bike without another word.

They kept moving. The afternoon stretched long and bright. Rolling hills gave way to flatter country, then sparse desert roads where heat shimmered in waves above the asphalt. Hours passed and slowly, against all logic, Drake found himself growing accustomed to the shape of their little convoy.

His bike in front, Donovan behind, and Ambrosia and the girl anchoring the rear. A strange sort of formation. Protective, almost. The thought made him snort under his breath inside the wind.

Ridiculous. He didn't need protecting. Didn't need company. Didn't need any of this and he sure as hell would never admit out loud that there was something oddly comforting about not being entirely alone on the road for once but somewhere deep down—
It was.

The realization sat quietly in his chest as dusk finally began bleeding across the horizon. Orange and violet painted the sky ahead, and when the glow of a roadside motel sign appeared in the distance, Drake knew he'd gone far enough for today.

He eased off the throttle and signaled toward the exit. Behind him, Donovan followed without question and farther back, Ambrosia's van drifted smoothly into line.

Like they'd all known exactly where they were going the whole time. Drake frowned at that thought as he pulled into the cracked parking lot. Whatever this was—It wasn't permanent. It wasn't real.

Just a stop along the way. Nothing more. That was what he told himself as he killed the engine and listened to the others pull in beside him and for reasons he refused to examine—The sound of them arriving made the empty motel lot feel a little less empty.

Chapter Nine

The days blurred together so completely that Drake eventually stopped trying to separate them.

At first, he'd kept track. He'd known roughly what week it was. Which state they'd crossed into. How long they'd stayed in one town before moving on to the next but somewhere along the line, that stopped mattering.

One week became another. Then a month passed. Then another. Seasons shifted around them without ceremony—heat giving way to cold, green leaves turning brittle and brown, snow falling in places Drake never planned to stop long enough to appreciate and still they kept moving.

Town to town. Motel to motel. Temporary jobs that paid in cash and asked few questions. Gas stations. Auto shops. Construction cleanup. Maintenance work.

Whatever Drake could pick up long enough to keep his savings growing before the road called again.

The rhythm became automatic. Wake. Work. Ride. Sleep, if sleep happened to come. Then repeat. Again,
and again and again. The road had always swallowed time for Drake but with Donovan, Ambrosia, and their daughter following him, it seemed to disappear entirely.

He didn't realize how much had passed until one afternoon when the truth hit him so suddenly it nearly stopped him cold.

It was at some forgettable little roadside motel somewhere in Arizona—or maybe New Mexico. Drake honestly couldn't say for sure. The heat had settled over the cracked pavement in thick waves, and he'd been halfway through changing the oil on his Harley in the motel lot while Ambrosia sat outside their room with the girl, working through some kind of reading lesson.

Drake wasn't paying attention. He'd long since learned how to let the sound of their voices drift into the background.

Then Ambrosia had sighed softly and said:

"No, Ally, sound it out."

Drake froze. The wrench stopped mid-turn in his hand.

Ally.

That was her name. The realization landed strangely hard. He'd been around this kid for a long time now and somehow he'd never actually known her name. He'd heard Donovan and Ambrosia speak to her a thousand times, probably. He just hadn't really listened but once he knew it, he couldn't unknow it.

Ally. It fit her somehow.

Bright and quick and impossible to ignore once you noticed her. He'd glanced over then and watched her wrinkle her nose in concentration as she sounded out whatever word was on the page.

She'd looked up suddenly and caught him staring. Instead of shrinking away or looking embarrassed like most kids would, she'd frowned.

"What?"

Drake had blinked. Then grunted and gone back to his bike. Behind him, he'd heard her mutter, "He's weird."
and to his own surprise—he laughed. A real laugh. Short and rough and rusty from lack of use, but unmistakably genuine. Ambrosia had stared at him like she'd just witnessed a miracle.

Ally had looked deeply offended that he was laughing at her and Drake had laughed harder.

That had been the first time. After that, Ally seemed to make it her mission to keep doing it. The kid had grown into a force of nature.

By the time Drake really looked at her—not just glanced in passing but actually looked—she wasn't the quiet little four-year-old clinging to Ambrosia's hand anymore.

She had to be at least eight now and that was when the realization unsettled him. Her black hair had grown longer, usually escaping whatever braid or ponytail Ambrosia had wrestled it into that morning.

Her green eyes—still impossible not to notice—were sharp with intelligence and endless opinion.

She talked constantly. About everything.

Why clouds moved. Why motorcycles were louder than vans. Why Donovan's dragon tattoo was "kind of creepy but also cool."

Why Drake never smiled. Why adults made dumb rules and why pancakes were objectively superior to waffles even though Donovan insisted otherwise and if she thought Drake wasn't listening, she'd simply repeat herself louder until he answered.

She was impossible. Exhausting. Too smart for her own good and somehow—Drake liked her. Not in any way he knew how to articulate. He just…did. The kid had a way of bulldozing straight through his walls simply because she didn't seem to realize they were there.

The first time she'd grabbed his cast-free hand months after it healed and dragged him toward a motel pool because she needed "a grown-up who isn't boring" to watch her jump in, he'd stared at her in disbelief.

Then followed anyway. Because saying no had somehow seemed harder.

That was what finally made it sink in. One evening, as Ally argued passionately over a board game in yet another motel room while Ambrosia laughed and Donovan looked deeply resigned to losing, Drake sat back in his chair and simply…noticed.

Noticed how much bigger she was. How easily she read now. How her front teeth had changed. How she'd grown inches taller. How comfortable she was around him and just like that, the truth hit him:

At least four years had passed. Four years. Drake sat very still as the realization settled over him.

Four entire years. Gone. He hadn't noticed. Hadn't marked birthdays or holidays or seasons. Time had simply slipped past while he kept moving forward, one empty road after another and suddenly—He was tired. Not physically. He could still outwork most men half his age.

No. This was deeper. A weariness that settled into his bones and stayed there. A realization that maybe he didn't want to do this forever.

The thought startled him. For nearly a decade, movement had been survival. Stopping meant vulnerability. Roots meant risk but now…now he found himself imagining something else.

Stillness. A garage, maybe. Somewhere he could finally tear his Harley apart and rebuild it properly instead of patching it together in motel lots. A place to save money without already planning his escape. A chance to actually think. To decide what came next instead of simply running toward whatever came after.

He glanced toward Ambrosia. She was sitting cross-legged on the motel bed flipping through TV channels, her face softer now than he remembered from the academy years. Older. Tired, too.

He could see it in her eyes. The constant moving wore on her in ways she rarely admitted and it had never even been her choice.

Donovan was the one who insisted they keep following Drake. Drake still didn't fully understand why. Four years and he still didn't know if Donovan was running from Helena, reporting to her, or trapped somewhere between both.

The uncertainty still unsettled him. Every so often, Drake caught Donovan watching the road too carefully, checking mirrors too often, tension settling into him at random sounds.

That wasn't guilt. That was fear. Whatever Helena's reach was, Donovan still believed it could find him.

Drake didn't know if he believed the same. As far as he could tell, Helena wasn't about to appear on some random motel doorstep in Kansas or Nevada or Texas and if she did—well he'd deal with her when the time came.

The thought no longer filled him with the same cold dread it once had. He wasn't twelve anymore. He wasn't trapped behind academy walls and Helena would learn that if she ever tried to drag him back. But for now—he was simply tired and for the first time in years, Drake let himself admit what he wanted.

He wanted to stop. Just for a while. Long enough to breathe. Long enough to figure out what kind of life came after all this endless motion. He didn't know where that place would be. Didn't know what it would look like. Didn't know if Donovan and Ambrosia would follow him there too but as Ally suddenly shouted in triumph over whatever game she'd just won and Donovan groaned dramatically enough to make her cackle with laughter—Drake found himself thinking that maybe if they did—he wouldn't mind.

Chapter Ten

Once Drake made the decision to stop moving for a while, everything seemed to fall into place faster than he expected.

Maybe because for the first time in years, he was actually looking for a place to stay instead of counting down the days until he could leave.

The thought still felt strange. Unnatural, almost.

Drake had spent so long living out of his backpack and the saddlebags on his Harley that the idea of having an actual address—even temporarily—felt foreign enough to make him uneasy but that unease was tempered by something else.

A quiet kind of relief he hadn't expected. For weeks after making the decision, he kept his eyes open whenever they rolled through towns that seemed decent enough. Somewhere small enough to stay under the radar, but large enough to have enough work to keep cash flowing in.

Nothing flashy or expensive. Just practical. Eventually, they found it. It was Donovan, of all people, who spotted the faded FOR SALE sign first.

They'd rolled into a quiet little town tucked against the edge of rolling hills and dry open country. The kind of place where people waved from porches and everyone probably knew everyone else's business by lunch.

Drake would normally have hated that but something about it felt…calm. Safe, maybe.

The duplex sat on a quiet side street lined with mature trees whose branches stretched over the cracked sidewalks like welcoming arms. It was older—probably built decades ago—and showed every year of it. The pale blue paint had faded badly in places, peeling near the shutters.

The porch steps sagged slightly to one side. Weeds had overtaken the flowerbeds, and one section of gutter hung loose enough to rattle when the wind caught it.

The roof looked solid enough, though and the foundation didn't seem compromised.

Drake could tell all that with one glance. Fixable. All of it. He liked that immediately because a fixer-upper meant leverage and leverage meant a lower price.

The owner had been an older man eager to offload it after his wife passed and his kids convinced him to move closer to family.

Drake saw the desperation there and haggled ruthlessly. By the end of the afternoon, after an hour of hard negotiation and enough cash placed on the table to make it clear he was serious, the duplex was his at a price low enough to leave him with enough savings to breathe.

When he stepped back outside with the paperwork in hand, Donovan was leaning against the van while Ambrosia stood nearby with Ally.

All three looked at him expectantly. Drake stared at the duplex for a long moment and then jerked his chin toward the larger side—the half with two bedrooms.

"You three can take that one."

Ambrosia blinked.

"What?"

Drake shrugged like it was obvious.

"Kid needs her own room."

For once, Donovan looked genuinely speechless. Ally, however, gasped loud enough to startle a bird out of the nearby tree.

“My own room?” Her eyes went huge.

Drake grunted.

“Yeah.”

Before he could brace himself, she launched at him. He barely caught her before she collided full-force into his ribs, her skinny arms wrapping around his middle.

“Thank you!”

Drake stiffened immediately.

He had no idea what to do with this. Physical affection wasn’t exactly something he knew how to process.
Awkwardly, after several painful seconds, he patted her head like she was some kind of stray dog.

“There. Alright. Enough.”

She laughed and let go, darting toward the duplex steps with enough excitement to nearly trip over herself.

Ambrosia was smiling. A real smile. Soft and warm in a way he rarely saw from her anymore.

“That was kind of you.”

Drake looked away immediately.

"Kid was getting too big to sleep in the same room as you two."

Ambrosia's smile widened because she knew exactly what he was doing—deflecting.

Donovan watched all of it quietly. There was something unreadable in his expression. Gratitude, maybe. Drake didn't want to examine it too closely.

The move-in itself took only two days. They didn't own much. Years on the road had a way of teaching you what mattered and what didn't.

A few bags of clothes. Books for Ally. Ambrosia's small collection of kitchen supplies she refused to part with. Donovan's battered tool case. Drake's own sparse belongings and enough motorcycle gear to rebuild half his Harley from scratch. That was about it.

By the second evening, they were settled enough to collapse into a tired silence broken only by Ally's delighted chatter as she bounced around her new room.

Drake stood in the doorway for a while watching her. She'd already claimed every inch of the place. Books stacked on the desk by the window. Her little stuffed animals lined neatly across the bed. A blanket Ambrosia had carried for years tucked carefully at the foot of the mattress.

She looked impossibly proud. Like she'd just been handed a castle. It hit Drake unexpectedly hard. He couldn't remember ever feeling that way about a room. About a home.

When he finally stepped back into his own half of the duplex, the silence waiting for him didn't feel lonely. That surprised him most of all. The place was simple.

One bedroom, a small living room and a kitchen that needed work. The bathroom faucet leaked. The flooring creaked. The walls needed paint. It was perfect. Work to do. Things to fix.

Something solid enough to keep his hands busy while his mind figured out what came next.

For the first time since his academy days, Drake unpacked fully. He put his clothes in drawers, set his tools in the small utility closet, and hung his leather jacket by the door instead of tossing it over a chair.

Small things. Normal things. The kind of things people did when they expected to stay. That first night, after everyone had settled, Drake sat alone on his small front porch. The summer air was warm and carried the scent of fresh-cut grass from somewhere nearby.

Through the shared wall, he could hear muffled laughter. Ally arguing with Donovan about bedtime. Ambrosia trying—and failing—not to laugh. It sounded…domestic. Normal. The kind of life Drake had spent years convincing himself he didn't want. He leaned back in the old porch chair and stared out at the quiet street.

No motel parking lot. No packed bags waiting by the door. No need to leave before dawn. Just a place to rest. A place to think. A place to breathe.

It wouldn't be permanent. He knew that. Sooner or later, the road would call again, or Helena would come, or Donovan's secrets would finally surface and ruin whatever strange peace they'd managed to build.

Drake wasn't naïve enough to believe otherwise but for now—for this moment—this would do and as the sounds of Ally's laughter drifted through the wall again, Drake realized something that unsettled him far more than any highway ever had.

For the first time in nearly a decade—he felt like he could relax, at least for a while.

It didn't take long for Drake to settle into a rhythm. That surprised him more than anything. For years, his life had been built around motion—constant, restless movement that never allowed enough stillness for roots to form. He'd convinced himself that was all he was capable of. That if he stopped for too long, the walls would close in and something terrible would eventually come for him the way it always had.

But this…This worked.

The days began early.

Drake usually woke before sunrise, not because he wanted to but because his body had long since forgotten how to sleep past dawn. Even on the rare nights where exhaustion dragged him under for more than four hours, it was never restful.

He'd wake tangled in sheets, his chest tight and damp with sweat, half-lost in whatever fractured nightmare Dragonfly Academy had dug into him all those years ago. The dreams were never the same.

Sometimes it was Helena's voice, cold and sharp, echoing down those endless sterile hallways. Sometimes it was the sound of fists meeting flesh. Sometimes it was nothing more than that awful crushing certainty that he was trapped again—that no matter how hard he fought, those walls would never let him leave.

Those were the worst ones. He'd wake gasping, his eyes wide in the dark, every muscle drawn taut for a fight that wasn't there and then he'd lie still in the flickering glow of whatever late-night infomercial the television had drifted to, waiting for his pulse to slow.

He always fell asleep with the TV on. The low murmur of voices helped drown out his own thoughts just enough to let sleep find him eventually.

By six, he was usually up and dressed, moving quietly through the duplex with practiced efficiency. Coffee. Boots. Leather jacket if the mornings were cold enough.

Then he was out the door. The local mechanic's shop had hired both him and Donovan almost immediately. The owner, Frank, was an older guy with grease permanently embedded in the lines of his hands and enough practical sense not to ask too many questions. He'd taken one look at Drake's Harley, then another at the way Drake handled an engine, and offered him a job before they'd even finished talking.

Donovan had followed naturally enough and somehow, against all logic, they worked well together. Not friends. Drake would never call them that but years of surviving Dragonfly Academy had left them with a strange, unspoken understanding of each other's habits.

They anticipated movements without thinking. Passed tools without asking. Worked side by side in easy silence broken only by occasional dry remarks or Donovan's muttered sarcasm.

Customers liked Drake because he rarely smiled and fixed things fast. They liked Donovan because he smiled enough for both of them. It worked.

The work kept Drake's hands busy and his mind quieter than it had been in years and his savings account—well, his lockbox hidden under the floorboards—was growing faster than he was spending it.

At home, Ambrosia had found her own rhythm too. She stayed with Ally, homeschooling her during the mornings and keeping their little half of the duplex running with a kind of quiet efficiency Drake had come to admire but unlike life on the road, staying put gave them opportunities.

There were neighborhood playgroups now. Library reading circles. Park meetups. Places where Ally could spend time with other children instead of being cooped up in vans and motel rooms.

Drake hadn't realized how badly the girl needed that until he saw her come home after her first playdate, breathless and bright-eyed, talking so fast no one could keep up. Apparently another little girl named Mia had strong opinions about dinosaurs and Ally had needed to "educate her extensively."

Drake had laughed hard enough to nearly choke on his coffee. Ally had looked deeply offended but then laughed too.

It was…good. Too good and that was what unsettled Drake most. He wanted to trust it. Wanted to believe this quiet little life they'd built could last but experience had taught him better.

Nothing good stayed. Not for him. That knowledge sat heavy in his chest no matter how normal things seemed. It kept him alert. Kept him from settling too deeply into comfort because comfort made people careless and careless people got hurt.

That was why, about a week after settling into this new rhythm, Drake found himself at the nearest bar on a Friday night. Not because he was unhappy but because something in him still resisted peace.

When life got too stable, some old instinct always made him restless. Like he needed to remind himself that this wasn't permanent.

That he was still Drake Rathburn. Still the man who left before roots could grow. So after work, after cleaning up and changing into dark jeans and a fitted black shirt that showed off the tattoos climbing his arms, he got on his bike and headed into town.

The bar was small and dimly lit, warm amber light spilling across polished wood and low conversation. The usual sort of place.

Not too crowded. Not too quiet. Perfect for what he wanted.

Company. Nothing more. No names that mattered. No attachment. Just enough distraction to scratch that old familiar itch.

He ordered whiskey and leaned against the bar, letting his eyes drift over the room. That was when he saw her. She sat alone at a small table near the back.

Blonde hair draped loosely over her shoulders, catching the low light in soft gold strands. Her hands were wrapped around a glass of soda, untouched except for the condensation dampening her fingers.

No alcohol. That was unusual here.

Something about the way she sat struck him too—too still somehow. Like she was trying to take up as little space as possible and when she looked up—Drake paused.

Hazel eyes met his. Soft, cautious, unexpectedly lovely. A strange flicker of familiarity hit him so suddenly it made his stomach tighten. For half a second, he thought he should know her.

Had met her somewhere. Seen those eyes before but the feeling vanished almost as quickly as it came, and Drake brushed it off.

Probably just some trick of memory. He crossed the room before he could think too much about it. The scrape of his boots against the floor made her startle slightly.

Not dramatically. Just enough to notice.

Her fingers tightened around the glass as she looked up at him. Up close, she was even prettier than he'd first thought. Young, maybe mid to late twenties. Delicate features.

A softness to her face that made her look almost fragile. Drake offered the same crooked smile that had gotten him into more beds than he could count. It came naturally. Easy charm over dangerous edges.

"Mind if I sit?"

She hesitated only a second and then gave a small nod.

He sat. She spoke softly when he asked her name.

"Catarina." Her voice was barely above the bar's low music.

Quiet. Measured. Like she'd learned not to waste words. Drake introduced himself and asked where she was from. Simple things.

She answered politely but sparingly, her hazel eyes watching him with careful attention. Most women would've filled the silences nervously. She didn't. She just sat there, composed and observant, and somehow that intrigued him more than easy conversation would have.

He kept the smile in place. Leaned in slightly. Let his voice lower. He knew exactly how to guide moments like this. It had become second nature years ago and sure enough, before long he asked the question he always eventually asked.

"Want to come home with me?"

Simple. Direct. No games.

Catarina studied him for a long moment. Something unreadable flickered behind those hazel eyes and then—She nodded.

Just like that. No hesitation or flirtatious teasing. Just quiet agreement. Something about it should have felt strange.

Instead, Drake simply stood and offered his hand. She took it. Her fingers were cool against his palm and together, they left the bar.

Outside, the night air was cool and still. Drake led her toward his Harley, already mentally preparing for another temporary distraction, another nameless night he'd forget by morning but as Catarina climbed on behind him and wrapped her arms carefully around his waist—That odd flicker of familiarity brushed against him again.

Stronger this time. Enough to make him glance back at her. Her hazel eyes met his in the dim light. Calm. Watching, waiting, and for reasons he couldn't explain—A faint unease settled in his chest.

Still, he said nothing. Just started the bike and drove them home.

Chapter Eleven

Drake barely made it through the front door before his hands were on her again.

The ride back to the duplex had left him wound tight in a different way than before, the cool night air and the feel of Catarina pressed against his back only sharpening the restless energy simmering beneath his skin.

The house was dark and quiet when they entered.

Donovan and Ambrosia's side of the duplex had long since gone silent, and the only sound in Drake's half was the low hum of the refrigerator and the faint creak of old floorboards beneath their feet.

Drake kicked the door shut behind them without bothering with the lights. The porch glow filtering through the blinds painted the room in muted gold and shadow.

Catarina stood near the door for a moment, watching him quietly. There was still something oddly restrained about her. Most women he brought home were easier to read. Flirtier. Bolder. Nervous in ways he understood but Catarina simply looked at him with those steady hazel eyes, calm and unreadable.

That strange flicker of unease brushed against him again. He ignored it. He stepped closer instead. Close enough to feel the warmth radiating from her body. Close enough to smell the faint trace of vanilla and cigarette smoke clinging to her hair from the bar.

His hand slid along her waist.

"You're quiet," he murmured.

A faint shrug.

"I don't talk much."

Her voice was soft enough that he almost didn't hear it. Drake gave a low hum of acknowledgment before leaning down and kissing her and just like that, the rest of the world disappeared.

He guided her backward through the narrow hallway toward his bedroom, never really breaking the kiss for more than a breath at a time.

His hands were rough and warm against her body, sliding over her hips, her back, the curve of her waist as he maneuvered them through the darkened space almost entirely by instinct.

The bedroom door bumped open against the wall. Moments later they collapsed onto the bed together, the mattress dipping sharply beneath their combined weight.

Drake landed above her, bracing himself on one arm as his mouth found hers again immediately.

The kiss deepened fast. Hungry. Desperate in a way that had less to do with desire and more to do with the constant restless ache living inside him. Catarina kissed him back, though there was hesitation in it at first. A softness. Like she was following his lead rather than losing herself in the moment.

Drake barely noticed. His hand slid into her hair as he tilted his head, urging her closer. When her lips remained closed, he pressed a little deeper, tongue brushing insistently against her mouth in silent encouragement. A quiet sound escaped her throat before she finally opened for him.

Then their tongues met. The kiss turned heated instantly. Drake exhaled sharply through his nose, his body settling heavier against hers as he lost himself in it.

Her fingers curled weakly against his shoulders. Still restrained, still oddly, and passive that nagging feeling returned. Something wasn't right. He couldn't place it. Couldn't define it but beneath the heat and adrenaline, some instinct kept scratching at the back of his mind.

Too quiet. Too compliant. Too distant somehow.

Drake ignored it anyway because thinking too hard was dangerous for him. Thinking led to memories. To doubts. To things he didn't want to feel. So instead he kissed her harder.

His rough hand slid along her side while his mouth moved against hers with growing urgency, only breaking away briefly every few moments for air before diving back in again.

The room filled with uneven breathing and the soft creak of the mattress beneath them. Outside, somewhere beyond the thin duplex walls, a dog barked faintly in the distance.

A car passed down the street. Normal sounds. Ordinary sounds but Drake barely heard any of it. He was too focused on drowning out his own thoughts. Catarina's hands finally moved more deliberately against him, though still carefully, almost cautiously, like she was learning him rather than simply reacting.

Drake's brow furrowed slightly against the kiss. Again—that feeling. Familiarity. Not with her exactly but with the moment. With the way she watched him even when they kissed. Like she was searching for something. It made his chest tighten unexpectedly. He pulled back just enough to breathe, their faces still inches apart.

For a second neither of them spoke. In the dimness, her hazel eyes looked almost golden. Steady on his. Not glazed with lust but with intent. Drake stared at her harder now, trying to place why that unsettled him so much. Then Catarina lifted one hand slowly and brushed her fingers against the smooth side of his bald head.

The touch was unexpectedly gentle and something about it made that uneasy feeling deepen instead of fade but before Drake could fully examine it, she leaned upward and kissed him again softly, drawing him back into the heat of the moment before he could think too much about why his instincts kept warning him that something about this night was wrong.

The room had grown warm, the air thick with the mingled scent of expensive bourbon and skin-warmed perfume. Outside, the city hummed its midnight song—distant sirens, the occasional rumble of a passing cab—but within these four walls, time had narrowed to nothing more than the space between their bodies.

Drake's hands moved with a practiced confidence, his fingers finding the delicate buttons of Catarina's silk blouse and releasing them one by one with a patience that belied the urgency thrumming through his veins. The fabric parted like water, revealing the pale expanse of her collarbone, the gentle swell of her breasts rising and falling with quickened breath. He traced the path of his progress with his mouth, following the trail of exposed skin with lips that knew exactly how much pressure to apply, exactly where to linger.

Catarina's fingers rested on his shoulder, neither pulling nor pushing, simply holding on as if anchoring herself to something solid in a world that had begun to tilt. When her blouse finally slipped from her shoulders and pooled on the floor beside them, Drake turned his attention to the clasp of her skirt, the zipper of his own trousers, the increasingly frantic shedding of barriers between them.

Clothes accumulated like shed skins across the room—her lace bra draped over a lampshade, his shirt crumpled against the baseboard, her panties catching on the edge of the nightstand before sliding to the carpet.

They tumbled onto the bed together, the mattress accepting their weight with a whisper of expensive linens. Drake positioned himself above her, taking a moment to appreciate the view—her blonde hair fanning across the white pillowcase, her lips parted and swollen from his kisses, her body arching toward him with an invitation that needed no words.

He entered her with a hard thrust, deliberately, and he expected the familiar response—the gasp of pleasure, the nails digging into his back, the encouraging roll of hips. Instead, Catarina's body went rigid beneath him. Her eyes squeezed shut, her jaw clenching as her teeth captured her bottom lip, whitening the flesh with the pressure of her bite. Her hands, which had been resting against his shoulders, suddenly moved to the sheets beside her, fingers twisting into the cheap cotton with a grip so tight her knuckles turned pale as bone.

Drake went absolutely still, his heart stuttering in his chest. The heat between them seemed to cool in an instant, replaced by the cold wash of concern.

"Hey," he whispered, his voice rough with restrained desire and sudden worry. "Hey, talk to me."

She didn't open her eyes. Didn't speak. Her breathing came in shallow, controlled sips through her nose, her chest barely rising.

Drake's mind raced through possibilities, each one landing like a stone in his gut. Had he misread her signals? Had he been too rough, too eager, too careless with his considerable size? He knew the feel of a virgin—he'd been with enough of them in his younger years to recognize that particular resistance, that untouched tightness that spoke of first times and trembling uncertainty. But Catarina didn't feel like that. There was no barrier to breach, no maidenhead resisting his advance. She simply felt... overwhelmed. Overfilled. As if his dimensions were stretching her to the very limit of her capacity, pressing against places that had never been touched so deeply.

He remained buried inside her, motionless, giving her body time to adjust to his presence, to soften around him, to accept the invasion and reshape itself to accommodate his length. The seconds stretched into minutes, marked only by the sound of their breathing and the distant wail of a car alarm on the street below.

Finally, her eyelids fluttered open. Her gaze found his, dark and unreadable, swimming with some emotion he couldn't quite name. She didn't speak. The silence between them felt heavy, charged with unspoken words.

"You good?" Drake asked, his thumb brushing gently against her cheekbone. She nodded, a small, tight movement that didn't quite reach her eyes.

"Did I hurt you?" The question came out softer than he intended, stripped of his usual bedroom confidence. Another shake of her head. Still, she said nothing.

Drake searched her face for the truth, finding only a mask of composure that seemed fragile, ready to crack. He wanted to ask more, to demand she tell him what she was feeling, what she was thinking, why she lay beneath him like a woman enduring something rather than enjoying it. But something in her silence stopped him—the set of her jaw, the way she refused to break eye contact, as if challenging him to continue or to withdraw.

He chose to continue, but with a gentleness that cost him. Every instinct screamed at him to move, to claim, to take what she had offered, but he ignored them all. Instead, he withdrew almost completely, feeling the wet heat of her surrounding just the tip of him, then pressed forward again with agonizing slowness. A gentle rocking motion, shallow and careful, treating her as if she were made of glass that might shatter beneath him.

A sound escaped her then—not quite a moan, more like a caught breath that had slipped past her defenses, involuntary and raw. It was small, barely audible, but Drake heard it. His lips curved into a grin against her shoulder, triumphant and relieved. That's it, he thought. That's what she needs. Slow. Gentle. Let her feel all of it without the rush.

He maintained his unhurried pace, each thrust deliberate and measured, angling his hips to drag against the places that made women gasp and clutch. He leaned down, capturing her mouth in a kiss that started tender and deepened as he felt her begin to respond. Her lips moved against his, hesitant at first, then with growing confidence. Her tongue met his, and he tasted the sweetness of the wine they'd shared earlier, the mint of her toothpaste, something uniquely her that he couldn't name but wanted to memorize.

She was kissing him back. Really kissing him. Her hands left the tortured sheets and found his back, her palms flat against his shoulder blades, pulling him closer. He felt the tension beginning to drain from her body, felt the muscles that had been rigid with strain beginning to soften, to welcome. It was working. She was relaxing into it, into him, her body finally accepting what he was giving and beginning to crave more.

Drake moved his mouth from her lips to her jaw, tracing the elegant line with open-mouthed kisses that left faint marks on her skin. He continued downward, finding the pulse point in her throat where her heartbeat fluttered like a trapped bird, laving it with his tongue before continuing his exploration. He wanted to know every inch of her, to map her body with his mouth and hands, to discover what made her sigh and what made her moan.

He shifted his weight to one elbow and reached up with his free hand to brush aside the curtain of blonde hair that had fallen across her neck and shoulder. The strands were silk against his fingers, catching the dim lamplight with auburn highlights he hadn't noticed before. He pushed the hair back, exposing the elegant column of her throat, the delicate shell of her ear, the smooth skin behind it where the neck curved into the skull—And froze.

There, inked into the pale flesh just behind her earlobe, no larger than a silver dollar, was a butterfly. Its wings were spread in mid-flight, rendered in shades of black and gray that gave it a three-dimensional quality, as if it might flutter away at any moment. The detail was exquisite—the veining in the wings, the delicate antennae, the suggestion of movement captured forever in skin.

Drake's blood turned to ice in his veins. He remained perfectly still, his body rigid above hers, his hand still tangled in her hair, his hips frozen mid-thrust. The tattoo stared back at him with its silent, permanent gaze, and suddenly everything made terrible, horrible sense.

The uneasy feeling that had been gnawing at the edges of his consciousness all evening—the sense that something was off, that the pieces didn't quite fit, that the woman beneath him was familiar in ways he couldn't quite place—crystallized into sharp, painful clarity.

He knew that tattoo. He'd seen it before, years ago, in a different lifetime, on a different girl who had laughed and called it her "secret wings." He'd traced it with his finger once, in a moment of tenderness he'd thought was love, had kissed that exact spot while whispering promises he'd been too young to keep.

Catarina hadn't moved. She lay beneath him, her eyes closed again, her face turned away as if she couldn't bear to watch his realization dawn. If she noticed that he'd stopped, that his body had gone cold and stiff inside her, she gave no sign. She simply waited, her chest rising and falling with shallow breaths, her hands resting now on his hips with a lightness that felt like goodbye.

Drake stared at the butterfly, at the small, permanent mark that changed everything, and felt the ground open up beneath him. He understood now why she'd been so quiet, why she'd gripped the sheets instead of him, why she'd closed her eyes and refused to speak. He understood the weight of what was happening between them, the collision of past and present, the secret she'd been keeping that had nothing to do with virginity and everything to do with history.

That was when he knew. That was when Drake understood why he'd had that uneasy feeling all night, why something in his gut had been screaming at him to stop, to look closer, to remember. The butterfly had been the key all along, hiding in plain sight, waiting for the moment when passion cleared enough for recognition to rush in.

And now that he knew, she was a butterfly.

Chapter Twelve

Drake stayed perfectly still.

The kiss had broken.

The heat that had filled the room moments ago seemed to evaporate, leaving behind a strange tension that settled heavily between them.

He hovered above Catarina, still buried deep inside her, one arm braced against the mattress, his eyes fixed on her face. The feeling he'd been trying to ignore was no longer a faint nagging sensation.

It was certainty.

His heartbeat slowed, his breathing steadied, and suddenly all he could see was the tiny details he should have noticed sooner.

The way she watched him. The way she'd barely spoken.

The strange familiarity that had tugged at him from the moment he'd seen her in the bar. Neither of them spoke for several long seconds until Catarina's quiet voice finally broke the silence.

"What's wrong?"

Drake held her gaze. For a moment he simply stared at her. Then he said the words that had suddenly become impossible to ignore.

"You're a butterfly."

The color drained from her face. That was answer enough. Drake rolled off her immediately and landed heavily on his back beside her.

The mattress shifted beneath their weight. The ceiling stared back at him. For several minutes neither of them moved and the room was silent except for the faint hum of the air conditioner and the distant bark of a dog somewhere outside.

Drake dragged a hand across his face. Of course it couldn't just be some random woman in a bar. Of course Helena somehow found a way back into his life. Again.

Eventually he sat up. The motion felt mechanical. Detached. He swung his legs over the edge of the bed and started looking for his clothes.

His boxers were crumpled near the foot of the mattress. He grabbed them and pulled them on without a word.
Behind him, Catarina slowly sat up. The blanket came with her, clutched tightly against her chest and chin like armor.

She looked frightened now. Small. Far younger than she had in the bar.

"I thought you knew..."

Her voice barely carried across the room. Drake turned toward her.

"I went five years without seeing or hearing from anyone from the academy." His voice was calm. "Then out of nowhere Donovan and Ambrosia show back up in my life."

He folded his arms across his chest.

"It hasn't exactly been bad having them around." That surprised him to admit aloud but it was true. "As strange as it is."

His eyes returned to hers.

"But now you." The words hung heavily. "A total stranger walks into my life and turns out to be from Butterfly."

He shook his head.

"I know that's not a coincidence." The room seemed to shrink around them. "So who sent you?"

Catarina's hands tightened on the blanket.

"And how did they know where I was?"

Silence. The fear in her eyes grew. Drake watched tears begin gathering along her lower lashes. No answer. His jaw tightened. A terrible suspicion surfaced. One that had been lurking in the back of his mind for years.

"Donovan."

The name came out low. Catarina flinched. Drake noticed immediately.

"Donovan is *still* communicating with Helena, isn't he?"

No response. His frustration surged.

"Isn't he?!"

The sudden sharpness in his voice made Catarina yelp. She immediately ducked beneath the blankets, disappearing completely.

The reaction hit Drake like a bucket of cold water. His shoulders slumped. Damn it. He exhaled heavily and rubbed the back of his neck.

"Catarina."

No response.

"It's okay."

The blanket shifted slightly.

"You don't have to be afraid of me." His voice softened considerably. "I'm not going to hurt you."

The room remained quiet. Eventually the blanket lowered enough for one frightened hazel eye to peek out.

Drake sighed.

"I know this wasn't your doing."

Looking at her now, she seemed terrified of disappointing someone. Terrified of making the wrong move. Terrified in a way that felt painfully familiar.

He remembered being that person. Back at the academy. Back when Helena's approval or disapproval could dictate every moment of a day.

"I just don't understand why Helena can't leave me alone."

His voice carried genuine exhaustion now.Slowly Catarina lowered the blanket. Not completely. Just enough for her face to become visible again.

Her eyes were red.

"I-I don't know." She looked down at her hands. "She just said you needed me."

Drake stared. Catarina swallowed hard.

"And she found out where you like to go."

The words sounded rehearsed. Like she'd repeated them to herself many times.

"She said I was supposed to wait." A tear finally escaped and slid down her cheek. "Every night."

Drake's expression darkened.

"Wait for me?"

Catarina nodded.

"Until you showed up." The room grew very still. "And I wasn't allowed to go home with anyone else."

Drake closed his eyes. For a second all he saw was Helena. Manipulating. Planning. Moving people around like pieces on a board. Even now. Even after all these years.

"I'm sorry." Catarina's voice cracked. "I really am."

Drake opened his eyes again. The apology wasn't necessary. If anything, he felt worse for her than for himself. Because whatever this was, she was trapped in it too.

Just like Donovan and Ambrosia were. He let out a long breath. Then pushed himself to his feet.

"Come on."

Catarina blinked.

"What?"

Drake grabbed a shirt from the floor and pulled it over his head.

"I'll make coffee." The simple normality of the statement seemed to confuse her. "In the morning we'll figure out what this is all about."

She stared.

"You still want me here?"

Drake snorted softly.

"Where else are you going to go tonight?"

That earned a tiny uncertain look. Not quite a smile but close. He headed toward the bedroom door then paused.

Without turning around he said quietly,

"I left the academy nine years ago." His hand rested on the doorframe. "And Helena needs to leave me alone once and for all."

Catarina looked at him then and the fear that had been in her eyes was gone. Instead there was something closer to hope.

As much as Drake hated the thought of it, he knew that he was going to have to confront Helena sooner rather than later or he would never have any peace.

Chapter Thirteen

The sun was barely beginning to rise when Drake loaded Catarina's small duffel bag onto the back seat of his Harley.

The town was still quiet. Most people were asleep. The streets were nearly empty except for the occasional delivery truck or early commuter heading to work.

Neither of them had gotten much sleep after their conversation. Drake had made coffee while Catarina had sat at his kitchen table wrapped in one of his old hoodies while she slowly explained pieces of her life. Not everything. There were still gaps. Still things she seemed afraid to say aloud but she'd told him enough.

Enough to make his stomach turn. Enough to make him hate the academies a little more.

Now they stood beside the motorcycle in the pale morning light. Catarina looked nervous. Not frightened. Not the way she'd looked the night before. This was different. This was uncertainty. The kind that came with standing on the edge of a completely new life.

"You sure about this?" Drake asked.

Catarina looked down at her hands and nodded.

"My parents..." Her voice trembled slightly. "I think about them all the time."

Drake stayed quiet. She swallowed hard.

"I don't even know if they still live in the same house."

The statement hit him harder than she probably realized. His thoughts immediately flashed back to his own hometown. To his father standing in the driveway. To the blond teenage boy learning everything Drake should have been learning.

He pushed the memory away. Catarina's situation was different. Unlike him, she hadn't chosen distance. She'd been robbed of it.

Kidnapped. A child stolen from her family and absorbed into the Butterfly Academy's twisted system.

The thought made his jaw tighten. Over the years he'd met plenty of kids who'd been sent there by parents who believed the lies of the evil ones running the academies.

But Catarina wasn't one of them. She'd never been abandoned. She'd been taken and she'd spent years too terrified to reach out even after becoming an adult. Not because she didn't want to but because they had made her believe she couldn't. The manipulation was infuriating.

Drake swung a leg over the Harley and handed her a helmet.

"Come on."

The ride to the bus station was quiet. Catarina sat behind him, holding on carefully while the motorcycle carried them through the awakening town. For once Drake didn't mind the silence. There wasn't really anything left to say.

The decision had already been made. The bus station sat near the edge of downtown. Nothing fancy. Just a squat concrete building with faded signs and a handful of buses arriving and departing throughout the day.

Drake parked near the entrance and killed the engine. The moment they stepped inside, Catarina's anxiety became obvious again.

She kept glancing around. Watching doors, watching people and watching exits. Years of conditioning didn't disappear overnight.

Drake understood that all too well. He walked beside her to the ticket counter.

"What city?" the clerk asked. Catarina hesitated. Then quietly gave the name of her hometown. The clerk typed for a moment.

Drake paid before Catarina could protest. The woman behind the counter printed the ticket and slid it across the desk.

"There you go."

Catarina stared down at the slip of paper. Her hands trembled as she accepted it. For a moment she simply stood there. Looking at it. Like she couldn't quite believe it was real.

A bus ticket. Something so ordinary yet somehow it represented freedom.

Drake gently nudged her shoulder.

"Looks like you're going home."

Her hazel eyes immediately filled with tears. This time they weren't tears of fear.

She laughed softly through them.

"I guess I am."

The announcement for boarding echoed through the station. Drake walked with her to the gate. The closer they got, the more emotional she seemed to become. By the time they reached the boarding line she looked like she might cry outright.

Drake rubbed the back of his neck awkwardly. He wasn't good at this sort of thing. Never had been but he tried anyway.

"Catarina."

She looked up.

"If anyone from the academies contacts you—"

"I have your number." She said.

"And you'll use it if you need to."

His voice was firm. Absolute.

For the first time since she'd met him, she seemed to truly believe him.

Drake continued.

"You're free now." The words settled heavily between them. "You go home."

He pointed toward the bus.

"You find your family." His expression softened slightly. "And you start your life over."

Fresh tears spilled down her cheeks. Drake ignored them. Not because he didn't care but because he knew she'd hate being fussed over.

"You'll be safe."

She nodded.

"I know."

"And nobody's coming after you."

Another nod. The boarding line began moving. People filed toward the bus. Families, college students, and travelers.

Normal people living normal lives. Something Catarina had never really been allowed to have.

She stepped forward then stopped. Before Drake could react, she suddenly leaned up and kissed his cheek. The gesture caught him completely off guard. He froze. Blinking. Catarina smiled through her tears. A genuine smile this time. The first one he'd really seen from her.

"Stay out of trouble." She said.

Drake actually choked. The sound was halfway between a cough and a laugh.

"That's probably not happening."

A tiny laugh escaped her. Then she turned and climbed aboard. Drake stood there watching through the windows as she found a seat. She waved.

He lifted a hand in return. A moment later the doors closed. The engine rumbled to life. The bus slowly pulled away from the station.

Drake remained where he was. Watching. Waiting. Until it disappeared completely from sight. Only then did he finally exhale. She had a chance now. A real one. More than most people from the academies ever got.

The thought stayed with him as he walked back to his motorcycle but once he climbed onto the Harley and started the engine, another thought quickly took its place.

Donovan.

The name settled heavily in his mind because Catarina's appearance wasn't random. None of it was. Helena had known where to find him. Known where he spent his evenings. Known enough to send Catarina directly into his path.

That information had come from somewhere and Drake was tired of pretending otherwise. For years he'd avoided the question. For years he'd let Donovan's presence linger around the edges of his life without forcing answers.

No more. He was done running from it. Done pretending it didn't matter. If he ever wanted peace in his life then he needed the truth. The Harley roared beneath him as he pulled out of the station parking lot.

He was going to make Donovan explain exactly why Helena still knew where Drake was after all these years. One way or another. The time for avoiding the inevitable was over.

Chapter Fourteen

Drake spent the entire ride home preparing himself for a confrontation.

For answers. For a fight if it came to that.

His Harley rumbled beneath him as he tore down familiar roads toward the duplex, his jaw clenched tight enough to ache. For years he'd ignored the questions. Ignored the inconsistencies. Ignored the nagging suspicion that Donovan knew far more than he admitted but after Catarina's confession, Drake was done pretending.

Helena had found him. Again and Drake knew that Donovan had to have been feeding her information. By the time he turned onto their street, his mind was already running through everything he wanted to say. Everything he wanted Donovan to explain.

Then he saw Ambrosia and immediately knew something was wrong. She was sitting on the front steps crying. Not the kind of tears someone sheds after an argument. She looked shattered. Completely broken.

Drake killed the engine before the motorcycle had fully stopped. The moment his boots hit the pavement, he was moving.

"Ambrosia?"

She startled violently at the sound of his voice. Her head snapped up. Her eyes were swollen red and mascara streaked her cheeks. For a second she looked so panicked Drake thought she might run.

"Easy." He slowed as he approached. "It's okay." Then he noticed the bruise. A dark mark spreading across her cheekbone.

Drake froze. Every muscle in his body tightened. The air seemed to leave his lungs. His eyes locked onto it.

"What happened?" His voice had gone dangerously quiet.

Ambrosia immediately looked away.

"Th-They took her..."

The words came out between ragged breaths. Drake frowned.

"They took who?"

For a second she couldn't answer. The tears came harder.

"Ally."

The name hit him like a punch. His stomach dropped.

"What?"

"Helena..." Ambrosia's voice broke. "And Darshire."

The names made Drake's blood run cold.

"They came and took her."

For several seconds Drake simply stared. His mind refusing to process what he'd heard. Then rage exploded through him. Pure. Immediate. Violent. His fists clenched so hard his knuckles cracked.

"What are you talking about?" The words came out sharp. "Where's Donovan?"

Ambrosia looked toward the duplex.

"He... he's inside."

That was all Drake needed. He turned and stormed toward the door. Behind him he heard Ambrosia call his name but he ignored her.

The front door slammed open hard enough to shake the frame. Inside, the living room was quiet and there on the couch sat Donovan. A beer bottle in one hand, looking calm.

For one brief second Drake thought he might actually kill him.

"Tell me what happened right now!"

The words thundered through the room. Donovan didn't flinch. Didn't even look surprised. He simply lifted the bottle and took another drink. Drake's temper snapped further.

"Donovan." Still nothing. "If you don't tell me what's going on right now—"

"Helena took Ally."

The interruption cut through the room like a knife. Drake stopped. Donovan set the beer bottle down. His unsettling red contacts reflected the afternoon light.

"She said it was time." His voice sounded hollow. "Time for Ally to enroll in Butterfly Academy."

Drake stared.

"No." The word escaped before he could stop it.

Donovan looked away.

"She said it was time for her training to begin."

Silence followed. Heavy. Oppressive. Then Drake exploded.

"And you just let them take her?"

The disbelief in his voice was overwhelming. He couldn't comprehend it. Could not process it. Donovan closed his eyes. His shoulders sagged.

"It was always going to happen."

The statement made Drake see red.

"What?"

"I did my best to keep her safe." Donovan's voice cracked slightly. "But—"

"But what?" Drake shouted. "What the hell does that mean?"

Donovan rubbed a hand across his face. The exhaustion there looked years old.

"It doesn't matter."

"Doesn't matter?" Drake laughed. A harsh, angry sound. "Your daughter was kidnapped!"

"Just leave it alone."

Drake stared at him. Then shook his head.

"Leave it alone?" His voice rose. "Leave it alone?" He took a step forward. "Hell no."

The words practically echoed.

"I'm going to get her back since you're apparently too weak to go after her yourself."

The moment the words left his mouth, Donovan stood.

"Drake." The warning in his voice was unusual. Serious. "Stop."

Drake turned toward him. Then Ambrosia appeared in the doorway. Her face was still wet with tears.

"We can't go after her."

Drake looked at her like she'd lost her mind.

"Yes we can." His fists clenched again. "Darshire might've been something when we were kids." His voice dripped contempt. "But he's no match for me now."

He meant it. The last time Drake had seen Helena's husband, he'd been younger, stronger, faster. Drake wasn't a scared twelve-year-old anymore. He wasn't trapped. He wasn't powerless. He could fight, he could hurt people, and he would if it got Ally back.

"It's not about that." Donovan's voice sounded strained.

Drake turned.

"What then?"

For the first time, Donovan looked genuinely shaken. Fear. Real fear. Not for himself. For Ally.

"If you go after her..." His throat tightened. The words seemed physically difficult to say.

"Helena will have Tony and Gunner..."

He stopped. Couldn't continue. His face twisted.

"She'll have them..." The rest wouldn't come.

Ambrosia closed her eyes. Then quietly finished for him.

"She'll have them welcome her to the Academy."

The room fell silent. Drake felt sick. Because he understood immediately. Understood exactly what they meant.

Tony and Gunner were former students from the first generation and they were known for their brutal punishment tactics and he knew what they did when tasked with "introducing" new arrivals. The same cycle. The same horrors.

The same abuse hidden beneath layers of manipulation and secrecy. The memories came flooding back. Things he'd spent years trying not to think about.

His stomach twisted violently.

"She's nine."

The words barely escaped him. Donovan nodded.

"She'll be fine for now."

Drake's eyes snapped toward him.

"Fine?"

"Helena promised Harold won't have her doing anything inappropriate yet." The word yet hung in the room. Poisonous. "If we cooperate."

Drake felt helplessness creeping in beneath the rage. A feeling he hated more than anything because he knew they were right. Charging in wouldn't work. Not against people like Helena. Not against the institutions George had built.

The academies survived because they were protected. Connected. Shielded by powerful people. People who benefited from what happened behind those walls. The authorities wouldn't help. The courts wouldn't help. Nobody ever did. That was how the academies survived generation after generation.

Drake hated it. Hated every second of it.

"So that's it?" His voice sounded hollow now. "We leave her there?" Neither answered. "So she can suffer the same way we did?"

Ambrosia broke first. Fresh tears rolled down her face. Donovan simply looked away.

"I'm sorry." The words sounded genuine. Broken. "I wish I had a solution."

Then Drake remembered Catarina. Remembered Helena knowing exactly where to find him. Remembered years of being followed. Watched. Tracked. The anger returned immediately.

"It's your fault."

Donovan stiffened.

"If you hadn't been reporting to Helena all these years—"

"I had to."

The interruption came fast. Desperate. Drake stared.

"What?"

"I had to."

"Why?"

Donovan looked away. Drake took a step closer.

"Why?" Still no answer. "What possible reason could justify this?"

Donovan sighed heavily. Years of exhaustion seemed to pour out of him.

"Just forget it."

Drake blinked.

"What?"

"Go live your life." Donovan's voice was flat. "We'll live ours."

"Donovan—"

"Forget you ever met Ally."

The words hit harder than a punch.

"No."

Drake shook his head immediately.

"No, I can't just—"

"Please."

The plea came from Ambrosia. She stepped forward. Her voice shattered.

"Please, Drake." Fresh tears fell. "It'll be worse for her if you don't."

The room went silent. Drake looked between them. Saw the fear. The hopelessness. The resignation and he realized neither of them believed Ally was coming home. Not anytime soon. Maybe not ever.

The realization hollowed him out. For several seconds he couldn't speak. Couldn't think. Couldn't breathe. Then he closed his eyes. Just for a moment. Trying to contain the rage threatening to consume him. When he opened them again, he didn't say another word.

There was nothing left to say. He turned and walked out. He crossed the yard, entered his side of the duplex, and slammed the door hard enough to rattle every window in the house. The sound echoed through the empty rooms.

Then silence returned. Drake stood alone in the middle of his living room. His chest rising and falling heavily. His fists still clenched. His mind replaying one thought over and over.

Nine years old. Ally was nine years old and Butterfly Academy had just claimed another child. This time someone he actually cared about. Drake hadn’t felt this truly powerless in years.

Drake stood in the center of his bedroom, breathing hard. The duplex felt too quiet. Every second that passed felt wrong. Somewhere out there, Ally was being driven toward the same nightmare that had stolen years of his life.

The same nightmare that had broken Donovan. Broken Ambrosia. Broken countless others. And everyone was expecting him to just sit here. To wait. To do nothing. His jaw clenched so hard it hurt.

"No." The word came out low and rough. "No damn way." He couldn't do it. Wouldn't do it. Every time he closed his eyes, he saw Ally's face. He saw her sitting at the kitchen table arguing over homework. He saw her proudly showing off books she'd read by herself. He heard her laughing when she beat Donovan at board games. He heard her calling him weird.

The kid was only nine. She should have been worried about playgrounds and cartoons and scraped knees. Not Helena. Not Darshire. Not Butterfly Academy. The thought made rage boil through him all over again. What infuriated him most wasn't even Helena.

Helena was exactly what she'd always been. A monster. A manipulative, calculating monster. No. What Drake couldn't understand was Donovan.

He paced the room. Back and forth. His boots thudded against the worn floorboards. How could he just let this happen? How could he sit there drinking a beer while his daughter was being taken? Drake couldn't make sense of it.

If Ally had been his child—his fists clenched. If Ally had been his daughter, he'd have fought until they killed him. He'd have burned the entire academy to the ground before handing her over.

Yet Donovan had sat there. Defeated. Accepting it. As if it were inevitable. As if there were no other choice. Maybe there wasn't. Maybe Donovan knew something Drake didn't.

But right now Drake didn't care. Because every instinct in his body screamed that Ally needed someone and if her father wasn't going to be that person—Then Drake would.

His fist slammed into the nightstand. The lamp rattled violently. The sharp pain shooting through his knuckles barely registered.

"Damn it!"

He spun around and yanked open the dresser drawers. Clothes were shoved into his backpack without any real organization.

Jeans. Shirts. Socks. Anything he thought he might need. The zipper strained as he crammed everything inside.

Then came the essentials. Cash. Every dollar he'd saved while working at the garage. The envelope disappeared into the bottom of the pack. A few motorcycle tools followed. Spare parts. A flashlight. A pocketknife. Everything he needed to survive on the road.

Because he already knew what this meant. His time here was over. The little slice of normal life he'd found had lasted longer than he ever expected. Long enough to make him almost believe he could stay.

Long enough to start imagining a future. A home. Roots. It had all been a lie or maybe just temporary. Either way, it was done now.

The moment Helena took Ally, everything changed. Drake pulled the backpack closed and slung it over his shoulder. The familiar weight settled against his back. Oddly comforting. Like slipping into an old skin.

The road again. The road always won but this time he wouldn't be riding alone. Not if he succeeded. Because once he got Ally back, he wasn't bringing her here. There would be no coming back.
No returning her to Donovan. No waiting for Helena to try again.

If Donovan wasn't willing to protect her—Then Drake would. He'd figure out the details later. Find somewhere safe. Somewhere hidden. Maybe another state. Maybe another country. It didn't matter. He'd make it work. He always did.

With one final glance around the room, he headed for the door. The small bedroom looked strangely empty now. A life abandoned. Again. Drake didn't hesitate. He marched through the duplex and out the front door. Then slammed it. Hard.

The sound exploded through the quiet neighborhood. The walls shook. The windows rattled. Some irrational part of him hoped Donovan heard it. Hoped he understood exactly how furious Drake was. Because right now, if Donovan stepped outside and tried to stop him—Drake wasn't sure how that conversation would end.

The cool evening air hit his face. His Harley sat waiting in the driveway. Faithful as ever. The one constant in his life. Drake crossed the yard in long strides. The backpack was secured quickly behind him. Straps tightened. Buckles checked. Everything locked down.

Then he swung his leg over the motorcycle. The familiar motion felt automatic. Natural. Like he'd never stopped traveling at all.

For a brief moment he looked toward the neighboring side of the duplex. The curtains were closed. No movement. No sign of Donovan or Ambrosia. Part of him wanted Donovan to come out.

Wanted him to give one good reason not to do this. One explanation that made sense. One truth that justified surrendering Ally but the door remained shut. The silence answered for him.

Drake's expression hardened.

"Fine." The word disappeared beneath the roar of the engine. The Harley came to life beneath him. The vibration traveled through the frame and into his bones. Power. Freedom. Purpose.

He knew exactly what he was going to do. Helena had taken Ally. Now Drake was going to take her back. No matter what stood in his way. No matter how many people he had to fight. No matter what secrets waited for him at Butterfly Academy.

He twisted the throttle. The motorcycle backed out of the driveway. Then surged forward. The duplex disappeared behind him. The town lights faded into the distance and Drake sped into the night, heading toward the place he'd spent years trying to forget.

Toward the academy. Toward a reckoning that had been building for nearly a decade. This time, he wasn't running away from it. This time, he was riding straight toward it.

Chapter Fifteen

The anger driving Drake forward burned hot enough that he barely noticed how many miles disappeared beneath his tires.

The Harley roared through the darkness, its headlight cutting a narrow path through the empty highway ahead.

His thoughts remained fixed on one thing. Ally. Every time he pictured her, the knot in his chest tightened.

Nine years old. Terrified. Being dragged toward Butterfly Academy.

Toward Helena. Toward the same nightmare that had stolen so much from all of them.

Drake gripped the handlebars harder.

He wasn't turning around. He didn't care what Donovan thought. He didn't care what Helena threatened. He wasn't abandoning Ally. Not without trying.

Hours passed before he finally noticed the fuel gauge hovering dangerously close to empty.

"Shit."

The curse disappeared into the wind. He glanced down. Not enough to keep going. Reluctantly, he began scanning for signs of civilization.

A few miles later, a gas station appeared beside the highway. The kind of lonely place that mostly catered to truckers and travelers passing through. A few pumps. A convenience store.

A flickering sign that looked like it hadn't been replaced in twenty years.

Perfect. Drake pulled into the lot and parked beside one of the pumps. The engine died. Suddenly everything felt too quiet. The realization hit him immediately.

His nerves prickled. Something wasn't right. He couldn't explain why. Years on the road had sharpened certain instincts.

The same instincts that had kept him alive through countless situations and right now every one of them was screaming.

Danger.

He ignored it at first. Maybe because his mind was elsewhere. Maybe because he was tired. Either way, he grabbed the nozzle and started filling the tank.

The gasoline flowed steadily. The sharp smell filled the air. Drake kept one eye on the dark parking lot. The other on the road.

Nothing. Everything appeared normal. Then he heard it. Footsteps approaching from behind.

Heavy. Purposeful. Not trying to hide. Not trying to sneak. The realization hit him instantly.

Bad. Before he could turn—A fist slammed into his jaw. The impact exploded across his face.

Pain shot through his head. His vision blurred briefly. The force sent him stumbling backward. The gas nozzle nearly slipped from his hand.

"What the—"

Drake caught himself before falling. His pulse surged. Adrenaline flooded his system. He straightened immediately.

Ready. His eyes snapped toward his attacker. Then recognition hit.

Braxton Jemenda.

Drake's expression darkened. Braxton stood a few feet away with his fists relaxed at his sides. He looked older now than Drake remembered.

Broader through the shoulders. More weathered but still unmistakably the same man.

A former Dragon. One of the boys from Drake's class. One of the academy's elite trainees. Someone Drake had never actually had a problem with which somehow made this worse.

"What the fuck was that for?" Drake rubbed his jaw. The spot already throbbed. Braxton didn't look particularly happy to be here.

If anything, he looked resigned.

"Helena." The single word answered everything. Drake laughed bitterly. "Helena wants to make sure you understand something."

Drake spat a little blood onto the pavement.

"Yeah?"

Braxton folded his arms.

"She wants you to know not to interfere." The words were calm. Measured. Like they had been rehearsed. "With Ally."

The mention of her name immediately reignited Drake's fury.

His jaw tightened as Braxton continued.

"She knew Donovan's warning wouldn't be enough."

Drake's eyes narrowed.

"What warning?"

"The one about what happens if you interfere."

Braxton's expression remained neutral.

"She knew you'd ignore it."

Drake took a step forward.

"Good."

Braxton sighed.

"That's why she sent us."

The word caught Drake's attention immediately. Us. His stomach sank. Slowly, he glanced around and realized that they weren't alone.

Figures emerged from the darkness surrounding the gas station. Some had been standing beside vehicles. Others stepped out from behind the convenience store. Several appeared near the edge of the parking lot. Watching. Waiting.

His heart sank. There were at least a dozen. Maybe more.

Dragons. Former students and classmates. Some faces he recognized immediately. Others had changed too much over the years but he knew what they were.

Knew what Helena had sent after him. The academy's attack dogs. The people trained specifically to enforce obedience. The people she trusted to handle problems.

People like Braxton. People who should have known better.

"Fuck."

The word escaped him quietly. A few of the Dragons shifted uneasily. Several avoided eye contact altogether. None of them looked eager. That stood out to Drake because this wasn't some group of loyal followers excited to carry out Helena's orders.

This looked more like obligation. Like people caught in a trap they couldn't escape. The realization didn't make him feel any better.

One of the Dragons stepped forward. A broad man Drake vaguely remembered from a class above his.

"Don't make this difficult."

Drake laughed. Actually laughed. The sound was harsh and humorless.

"Too late."

His backpack remained secured to the Harley. His bike sat behind him. The road ahead blocked. The road behind blocked too.

A trap. A deliberate one. Helena had known exactly where he would stop. Exactly what route he would take. Exactly how he'd react.

That realization infuriated him more than the punch. Braxton shook his head.

"Drake." His voice carried something almost sympathetic. "Just go home."

"No."

"She's not your kid." The words landed like gasoline on a fire.

Drake's eyes hardened instantly.

"No."

Braxton exhaled.

"Then don't say we didn't warn you."

Silence settled over the parking lot. The distant hum of traffic echoed across the highway. The gas pump clicked behind Drake. Tank full. Fueling complete. The sound seemed absurdly normal considering what was happening.

Drake rolled his shoulders once. Then twice loosening them. His jaw still hurt. His knuckles flexed. The old familiar feeling settled into place. The same feeling he'd carried into countless fights growing up.

The same feeling he'd learned at Dragonfly. Pain was coming.

He accepted that but if Helena thought he was just going to roll over and surrender—she hadn't learned a damn thing about him.

Drake straightened fully. The parking lot lights cast harsh shadows across the pavement. Around him, the Dragons began spreading out creating a circle and cutting off escape.

A dozen trained fighters against one man. The odds were terrible. Drake knew it. Braxton knew it. Everyone standing there knew it but Drake had never been particularly concerned with odds.

His green eyes swept across the gathering faces. Then settled on Braxton.

"Tell Helena something for me."

Braxton's expression tightened. Drake cracked his sore jaw then smiled. A dangerous smile. The kind that never ended well.

"I'm not twelve anymore."

The words hung in the air. Then Drake planted his feet firmly on the pavement, raised his fists, and prepared to make every one of them earn whatever message Helena wanted delivered.

Chapter Sixteen

Drake groaned as something cold pressed against the side of his face.

The chill bit into the rapidly swelling bruise on his cheek, making him flinch before he was fully awake.

He cracked one eye open. Everything was blurry.

Fluorescent lights buzzed overhead, painfully bright against the pounding in his skull. Shelves lined with chips, candy bars, and rows of motor oil slowly came into focus as his vision steadied.

He blinked several times. The smell of stale coffee and gasoline hung in thc air. A convenience store.

He frowned. Why?...then it came rushing back.

The gas station, Braxton, the punch, the circle of Dragons closing in around him, and the fight.

He remembered throwing the first punch after Braxton's warning. Remembered dropping one of the men with a hard elbow before another had tackled him from behind.

He remembered fists. Boots. Someone driving a knee into his ribs. He'd gotten back to his feet more than once. He always did but there had simply been too many of them.

Then...a sharp burning pain in his side. A knife. After that...nothing.

Drake sucked in a careful breath as the memories settled into place. His entire body protested. His jaw throbbed. His ribs felt bruised. Every muscle ached.

"You awake?"

The voice pulled his attention away from his thoughts. A middle-aged convenience store clerk crouched beside him, still holding the plastic bag of ice against Drake's cheek.

The man's face was lined with concern.

"You gave me a scare."

Drake slowly pushed himself more upright in the chair. His head swam immediately. He closed his eyes until the dizziness eased.

"I'm fine." His voice came out rough. Barely more than a mutter. "Nothing for you to worry about."

The clerk raised an eyebrow.

"No?" He gestured toward Drake's side. "What about the fact that you're bleeding?"

Drake looked down. Only then did he notice the dark stain spreading across the front of his gray T-shirt. It had soaked through the fabric near his right side and continued creeping outward.

His expression tightened. He still couldn't really feel it. Shock, probably. Adrenaline but he knew exactly what it was. Knife wound.

He lifted the edge of the shirt carefully. Sure enough, blood continued seeping steadily from a slash just below his ribs. It wasn't gushing which was good but it definitely wasn't stopping either.

Drake let the shirt fall again.

"I don't suppose you know how to stitch cuts?"

The clerk looked horrified.

"No." He answered immediately. "I absolutely do not."

Drake sighed. Figured.

"The ambulance is already on the way." The clerk folded his arms. "They're only a few minutes out."

Drake looked toward the front windows. His Harley still stood beside the pump outside. At least they hadn't taken the bike.

Small victory.

"Just keep pressure on it until they get here." The clerk reached behind the counter, grabbed a clean dish towel, and handed it over. "It doesn't look too deep." He hesitated. "But it definitely needs stitches."

Drake accepted the towel with a quiet grunt. He folded it against the wound, pressing firmly. The pressure immediately made the pain flare. He hissed through his teeth.

"There it is," he muttered. The feeling had finally caught up.

The clerk offered an awkward smile.

"Guess the adrenaline's wearing off."

"Yeah."

Drake leaned back again, letting his head rest against the wall behind him. This wasn't how tonight was supposed to go. He should've been halfway to Butterfly Academy by now. Instead...he'd been beaten bloody and stabbed.

Exactly what Helena wanted. He closed his eyes briefly. She hadn't sent Braxton and the others to kill him. If she'd wanted him dead, twelve trained Dragons would've made sure he never got back up.

No. This had been a message. A warning to stay away and don't interfere. Leave Ally where she is.

His jaw tightened. Not a chance but he knew something now that he hadn't wanted to admit before. He wasn't getting Ally out alone.

The attack had made that painfully clear. If Helena could organize an ambush before he even reached the academy...then she'd be expecting him every step of the way.

He needed another plan. People. Information. Something. Anything. His thoughts drifted to Ally. He pictured her sitting frightened in some unfamiliar dormitory.

Wondering where her parents were. Wondering if anyone was coming. The image twisted something inside his chest.

He lowered his head slightly.

"Just hang in there, Ally." His voice was barely audible. "I'm coming for you soon."

The words escaped before he realized he'd spoken them aloud. The clerk looked over curiously.

"Who's Ally?" Drake didn't answer. "And...who are you talking to?"

For several seconds Drake simply stared at the floor. Then he shook his head.

"No one." His voice was quiet. "Just..." He adjusted the towel against the wound again. "Do whatever you do." He forced a tired breath from his lungs. "I'll be out of here soon."

The clerk looked like he wanted to ask more questions but he nodded instead.

"Alright."

He stood and headed back behind the register, giving Drake a little space while still keeping an eye on him. The convenience store settled back into an uneasy silence. Only the buzzing lights, humming refrigerators, and distant traffic broke it.

Drake leaned his head back against the wall again. His side throbbed with every heartbeat. His cheek continued swelling beneath the melting bag of ice. He felt exhausted. Frustrated. Angrier than ever but beneath all of that...determined.

Helena had won tonight. There was no denying it. She'd stopped him. She'd forced him off the road. She'd proven she could still reach him whenever she wanted.

Drake hated every second of it. He let out another long, weary sigh. For now, he didn't have much choice. He'd let the paramedics patch him up. Let the doctors stitch the knife wound closed.

Then he'd start over.

Because one thing had become painfully clear. Charging blindly toward Butterfly Academy wasn't going to save Ally.

If he was going to bring her home...he was going to need a plan and this time—he intended to make sure Helena never saw it coming.

The hospital automatic doors slid open behind Drake as he stepped into the cool evening air. His side immediately protested.

The fresh stitches beneath the bandage pulled painfully with every movement, reminding him that he had been lucky. A few inches in another direction and the knife could have done far more damage.

The doctor had been very clear.

"Take it easy for a couple of weeks, don't lift anything heavy, take the pain medication as prescribed, and come back immediately if the wound starts bleeding through the bandage."

Drake had simply nodded through the entire lecture. He had no intention of following most of it. The small white prescription bottle rattled in his pocket as he climbed into the Uber waiting outside.

The driver glanced at him through the mirror.

"Hospital discharge?"

"Yeah."

"You alright?"

"I'll live."

The driver took the hint and didn't ask anything else. The ride back to the gas station was quiet. Streetlights drifted past the windows while Drake rested his forehead against the cool glass.

His body ached. His jaw was swollen purple from Braxton's punch. Several bruises had already begun blooming across his ribs and shoulders. Every bump in the road tugged at the stitches in his side.

He hated feeling weak. He hated sitting still even more. Twenty minutes later the car pulled into the familiar gas station parking lot.

Drake climbed out carefully, trying not to aggravate the wound.

The clerk spotted him immediately through the front window. A relieved smile crossed the man's face as he hurried outside.

"Hey."

"Told you I'd be back."

The clerk looked him over.

"You look a little better."

"I don't feel better." The clerk reached into his pocket and produced a key. "I moved your bike around back."

Drake raised an eyebrow.

"Didn't think it'd be a good idea leaving it sitting by the pumps overnight." He gestured toward the alley behind the building. "Figured somebody might decide it looked expensive."

Drake nodded appreciatively.

"Thanks."

The clerk shrugged.

"It would've been a shame if somebody stole it after everything else."

Together they walked around the building. There sat the Harley. Untouched. Seeing it brought an unexpected sense of relief.

It had been the one constant companion in his life for years. He rested a hand on the handlebars.

"Thanks for looking after her."

"No problem."

Drake carefully untied his backpack from the rear rack and checked its contents. Everything was still there. His tools. His spare clothes. The envelope of cash.

Nothing missing. He secured everything again before swinging a leg over the motorcycle. The movement pulled sharply against the stitches.

"Son of a..." He winced loudly.

The clerk folded his arms.

"You sure you should be riding?"

Drake adjusted himself in the seat.

"I'll be fine."

"You just got stabbed."

“So…”

"And the doctor let you leave?"

"Barely."

The clerk laughed quietly.

"I've got pain pills."

"That doesn't exactly make me feel better."

Drake smirked for the first time in what felt like days. The clerk remained standing beside the bike.

"I don't know what kind of trouble you're mixed-up in..." Drake looked at him. “But I hope you come out the other side."

The simple sincerity caught him off guard. For a second he didn't know what to say. Then he simply nodded.

"Thanks." He thumbed the starter. The Harley rumbled to life beneath him. The familiar vibration settled through his body.

Despite the pain...despite everything...it still felt like home. He pulled away from the station without another word. Soon the highway stretched endlessly before him once again.

The fading afternoon sun painted the horizon orange while the wind tugged at his clothes. His thoughts drifted back to the duplex.

It hadn't been much. An old fixer-upper split down the middle. Leaky pipes, crooked floors, and drafty windows but it had been home.

A place he'd actually unpacked. A place where he'd fallen into a routine. Working at the garage beside Donovan. Coming home every evening. Listening to Ally chatter endlessly about whatever book she'd been reading that day.

Watching Ambrosia slowly become comfortable enough to smile again. He hadn't realized how much he'd grown accustomed to it until it was gone. He'd even miss Donovan. As angry as he still was.

As much as he couldn't understand the man's choices. Donovan had become part of his everyday life. And Ambrosia...she'd always treated him with kindness despite everything they'd all survived.

Leaving them behind hurt more than he wanted to admit but Ally needed him. That fact outweighed everything else.

He twisted the throttle slightly as the motorcycle gained speed.

He couldn't rescue her alone. Braxton and the Dragons had already proven that. If Helena could assemble that many trained fighters just to stop one man…then storming the Academy by himself would be suicide.

No. He needed help. Real help. People willing to fight. People who didn't mind getting hurt. People who wouldn't walk away when things got ugly. The question was…where did someone even find men like that?

The thought stayed with him for miles. Then another idea slowly formed. At first it was only a whisper.

Small. Almost ridiculous.

He frowned. If he was going to risk everything...if he was going to build a team...if he was going to fight his way into Butterfly Academy...why stop at Ally?

His grip tightened around the handlebars. There were dozens of children inside those walls. Maybe hundreds.

Some were there because they had been abandoned. Others because they had been manipulated. Some, like Catarina...had been kidnapped outright. Every one of them deserved freedom.

The realization struck him with surprising force.

Why save one child...When he could try to save them all?

The idea was impossible. Dangerous. Maybe even insane. It would require planning unlike anything he'd ever attempted.

People. Resources, vehicles, safe places for rescued children, evidence and away to expose institutions that had spent decades hiding behind powerful friends and carefully crafted lies.

It would take more than muscle. It would take an army. Drake couldn't help smiling despite the pain.

For years he'd wandered the country without purpose. Simply surviving. Simply existing. Now, since walking out of Dragonfly Academy nine years earlier, he finally had something worth fighting for.

The Academies had stolen enough lives. They had stolen enough childhoods. They had been allowed to exist far longer than they ever should have.

Someone had to put an end to them. Someone had to be willing to stand between those children and the monsters waiting behind those gates.

The wind rushed around him as the Harley thundered farther down the highway. Drake's destination was still unknown but his purpose no longer was.

If no one else was going to destroy the Academies...then he would. No matter how long it took. No matter what it cost.

He would come back for Ally and when he did, he intended to tear the entire system down around Helena's ears.

Chapter Seventeen

Drake rode until the afternoon faded into evening, the miles disappearing beneath the tires of his Harley without meaning anything.

He hadn't chosen a destination. He hadn't even looked at a map. He simply followed whichever road felt right at the time, hoping that somewhere along the way an answer would come to him.

It never did. The steady rumble of the motorcycle gave him too much time to think. Every plan he came up with seemed to fall apart before it was fully formed.

He couldn't march into the academies alone. He couldn't go to the authorities. He couldn't ask Donovan for help. Even now Drake still didn't understand what held the other man back.

Fear. Loyalty. Blackmail. Whatever it was, Donovan had accepted that Ally was gone.

Drake refused to. Still, rescuing one little girl was one thing. Destroying the academies…that was something else entirely.

He needed people. Not just people. Fighters. Men and women willing to risk everything. People who wouldn't turn around the moment things became dangerous.

The problem was, where did someone even find people like that? He had spent nearly a decade avoiding attachments.

Avoiding friendships. Avoiding putting down roots. Now those choices were catching up with him. He had no one to call. No one to trust.

The realization settled heavily on his shoulders. By the time the sun had almost disappeared below the horizon, exhaustion was beginning to overtake him.

His side throbbed beneath the fresh stitches every time he shifted his weight. The pain medication from the hospital had dulled the ache somewhat, but it hadn't made it disappear.

He spotted a small roadside motel ahead. The faded neon sign buzzed lazily, announcing vacancies. It would do.

Drake pulled into the parking lot and parked near the end of the row of rooms. After paying for a single night, he dug through the backpack, searching for the one thing he wanted more than sleep.

"C'mon..." His fingers brushed against a crushed pack of cigarettes. "There you are." He fished out the pack and his lighter.

Before he could light one, raised voices echoed across the parking lot.

"What the hell, Hudson!"

Drake looked up. One of the nearby motel room doors burst open. Two young men stumbled backward into the parking lot, nearly tripping over one another as they fought to regain their balance.

"Son of a bitch!" One of them straightened his leather jacket with an irritated growl. The back immediately caught Drake's attention.

STRAY SONS.

A motorcycle club. Drake casually glanced around the parking lot. Sure enough, three motorcycles sat parked together only a few spaces away. Well maintained. Travel-worn. The kind of bikes that had seen countless highways.

Another figure appeared in the doorway. This one had wavy flame-red hair and an infuriatingly smug grin. A young scantily clad woman clung affectionately to his arm.

"You always do this, Hudson!" the light-brown-haired biker shouted.

Hudson only shrugged.

"Relax."

"You say that every damn time!"

Another man appeared behind him. He had black hair, several healing tattoos covering both arms and disappearing beneath his shirt collar.

He looked thoroughly exhausted.

"Fucking hell, Hudson." He rubbed a hand through his hair. "We finally get a room with an actual bed and you throw us out."

Hudson grinned wider.

"Shut up." He wrapped an arm around the woman beside him. "Sally here isn't staying all night."

The other two groaned loudly.

"Sure she isn't," the tattooed man muttered.

Hudson ignored them. The door closed. A second later the lock clicked.

Silence. The brown-haired biker stared at the door in disbelief.

"I'd like to kick it down and throw him out."

"I wouldn't." The tattooed man folded his arms. "If you do..." He smirked despite himself. "You're liable to see a whole lot more of Hudson than you ever wanted."

The brown-haired biker's face twisted.

"Fuck..." He dragged a hand down his face. "I'm going to get us some burgers." He pointed dramatically toward the closed motel room. "He'd better be done by the time I get back."

Without another word, he stomped toward the nearby fast-food restaurant.

Drake couldn't help the small chuckle that escaped him. He finally lit his cigarette and leaned comfortably against his Harley. The first drag settled his nerves almost instantly. A few moments later he noticed the tattooed biker walking his way.

"You mind if I bum one?"

Drake simply held out the pack. The young man slid one free.

"Thanks."

Drake flicked the lighter open. The biker leaned in, lit the cigarette, and took a long grateful drag before exhaling toward the darkening sky.

"Been one of those days?"

Drake asked. The man laughed tiredly.

"You could say that." He motioned toward Hudson's room. "That's just Hudson being Hudson."

Drake raised an eyebrow.

"We're usually too broke to afford motel rooms." The biker shrugged. "So whenever we actually get one, we've got to decide who gets the bed."

Drake nodded.

"But then Hudson meets some girl in a bar..." Another long drag. "Brings her back to get laid..." He pointed toward the closed door. "And Cullen and I get kicked outside."

Drake smirked.

"By the time he's done..." The biker shuddered dramatically. "Neither of us wants anything to do with that mattress."

That earned a genuine laugh from Drake.

"I suppose that's fair."

"I'm Viper." He extended a hand. Drake shook it.

"Drake."

Viper studied him for a moment.

"So what's your story?"

Drake looked down the empty highway.

"Just traveling."

That was all he offered. He wasn't ready to explain the academies, Ally or Helena. Viper seemed to recognize that there was more to the story but didn't push.

Instead Drake nodded toward the jackets.

"Stray Sons your club?"

Viper chuckled.

"Club's a generous word."

Drake looked back at him.

"It's really just the three of us." He pointed toward the burger restaurant. "Cullen." Then toward Hudson's room. "Hudson and me, we don’t have a clubhouse or territory, no big family backing us." Viper explained. So we just ride, work odd jobs, and try not to starve."

Drake found himself nodding. It sounded strangely familiar.

"You're welcome to use my room."

Viper blinked.

"What?"

"I don't sleep much." Drake shrugged. "You and Cullen can have the bed."

Viper looked him over carefully. Then shook his head.

"Nah, you need it more."

"I'm fine."

"You don't look fine."

Drake opened his mouth to argue when Viper reached out suddenly and poked him lightly in the side. Right where the old red stain and the stitches were.

Drake hissed through clenched teeth.

"Son of a—" He instinctively grabbed at the wound.

When Viper pulled his finger back, it came away smeared with fresh blood. Both men stared at it.

"Well..." Viper deadpanned. "That's probably not supposed to happen."

Drake looked down. A fresh red stain was slowly spreading through the bandage beneath his shirt. He cursed under his breath.

"I think..." He winced. "I might've pulled the stitches riding."

Viper folded his arms.

"You need that looked at."

"More like restitched." Drake sighed. "And before you suggest it, I'm not going back to the hospital."

Viper laughed.

"I wasn't." He nodded toward the fast-food restaurant. "Cullen can sew."

Drake looked skeptical.

"Cullen stitched our club patches onto our jackets." Viper grinned. "Steadiest hands out of the three of us."

Drake raised an eyebrow.

"That's your recommendation?"

"It's the only one you've got."

Despite himself, Drake laughed.

"I guess I'll have to settle for that."

Viper smiled.

"Cullen will be back in a few minutes." He crushed his cigarette beneath his boot. "Come on." He nodded toward Drake's motel room. "Let's get you sitting down before you fall over trying to act tough."

Drake rolled his eyes.

"I ain't falling over."

"You were bleeding through your bandage and didn't even notice."

"Fair point..."

Drake dropped his own cigarette to the pavement and ground it out beneath his heel. Together they walked toward his room and Drake found himself talking to someone without suspicion hanging over every word.

He didn't know it yet, but as he unlocked the motel room door and stepped inside beside Viper, fate had quietly placed the first piece of his impossible plan directly in his path.

Drake sucked in a sharp breath through his teeth as Cullen carefully pushed the needle through the edges of the wound.

"Easy," Cullen muttered. "Try not to move."

"I'm trying," Drake grumbled, gripping the edge of the motel mattress until his knuckles turned white.

The three of them had made a quick trip to the nearest Walgreens after Viper noticed the blood soaking through Drake's bandage. They hadn't been able to buy proper medical supplies, but they'd gathered enough to clean the wound and hopefully keep it closed until it had a chance to heal.

A bottle of peroxide sat open on the nightstand beside a pile of bloodstained cotton balls. The sharp chemical smell filled the room.

Cullen had sterilized the curved sewing needle as best he could before threading it with heavy-duty black thread from a small travel sewing kit he'd insisted on buying.

It certainly wasn't hospital quality but it was all they had. Drake hissed as another stitch pulled tight.

"Sorry," Cullen said without looking up. His hands remained surprisingly steady. "I'd rather this hurt now than split open again tomorrow."

"I know."

Drake leaned his head back against the wall and forced himself to stay still. His side burned with every pass of the needle. The pain medication the hospital had prescribed had dulled the ache earlier, but it wasn't nearly enough to make this pleasant.

Viper leaned against the dresser, arms folded across his chest while watching Cullen work.

"I still think you're crazy for leaving the hospital."

Drake snorted.

"I wasn't sticking around there."

"You got stabbed.”

"Yep."

"You should've let a doctor deal with it."

"I've had enough hospitals for one week."

Viper chuckled quietly.

"Fair enough, I hate hospitals too."

Cullen tied off another stitch before examining his work.

"This probably won't hold forever."

Drake looked down.

"What do you mean?"

Cullen clipped the excess thread.

"This isn't medical thread." He gestured toward the sewing kit. "It's just heavy-duty sewing thread." He shrugged apologetically. "It's strong enough to keep the wound closed for now." He looked Drake squarely in the eye. "But if you go wrestling somebody or riding that motorcycle like a maniac you're probably going to tear it open again."

Drake gave a dry laugh.

"So don't move around much."

"Exactly."

"I'll do my best."

"I somehow doubt that."

That earned a grin from Viper.

"I think that's the smartest thing you've said all night."

Drake rolled his eyes.

"You two done making fun of me?"

"Not even close."

Cullen carefully cleaned away the remaining blood around the stitches before placing a fresh bandage over the wound.

"There." He pressed gently around the edges to make sure it stayed in place. "That should do."

Drake looked down at the neat white bandage.

"Appreciate it."

"No problem."

The used cotton balls, empty peroxide bottle, wrappers, and bloody gauze were gathered into a plastic shopping bag. Viper tied the handles together before tossing it into the trash can outside the motel room. When he came back inside, Drake looked around the small room.

The single bed took up nearly half the space. The television sat atop a scarred wooden dresser. A tiny mini fridge hummed quietly in the corner. Nothing fancy. Just another roadside motel.

He looked between the two younger bikers.

"You guys sure you don't want this bed?"

Viper laughed.

"You already offered once."

"I'm offering again." Drake nodded toward the wall separating his room from Hudson's. "Your friend's probably going to be occupied for a while."

As if on cue, a muffled thump echoed through the wall. The three men froze. Another thump. Then laughter. Cullen groaned dramatically.

"I swear he plans this."

Drake couldn't help laughing. Viper buried his face in one hand.

"Every damn time."

Cullen looked toward the television.

"I heard there's a boxing match on HBO tonight." He glanced at the others. "We could just hang out in here until Hudson's... finished." The brief pause before the last word made both Drake and Viper laugh.

"Yeah." Viper nodded. "Why not?" He walked over to the mini fridge and opened it. A six pack of beer sat inside. He tossed one bottle to Drake. Another to Cullen. Then twisted the cap off his own.

The bottles clinked together.

"To temporary roommates."

Drake smiled faintly.

"I'll drink to that."

The television flickered to life. A boxing ring filled the screen as commentators discussed the upcoming main event. The three of them settled onto the bed, shoulder to shoulder, balancing their beers while the introductions played.

"So who you got?" Cullen asked.

"The guy in blue trunks," Drake answered. "He looks quicker."

Viper shook his head.

"No chance, the bigger guy's going to wear him down."

"You just like heavyweights."

"They hit harder."

"They're slower."

"They don't have to be fast if the other guy walks into one punch."

The opening bell rang. All three fell silent. The smaller fighter immediately began circling the ring.

"Told you," Drake said. "Too quick."

"Just wait." Viper took another drink.

Halfway through the second round, the larger boxer landed a crushing right hook that dropped his opponent to the canvas.

Viper pointed triumphantly at the television.

"What'd I say?"

Drake laughed.

"Alright, you got me."

Cullen grinned.

"I think you're both wrong."

The two other men looked at him.

"The smaller guy's getting back up."

Sure enough, he beat the count. The match continued.

Before long all three of them were arguing good-naturedly over every punch, every missed opportunity, and every questionable decision from the referee.

Drake found himself laughing. Really laughing. It caught him off guard. *When was the last time he'd done that?* Not a forced chuckle. Not bitter sarcasm. An actual laugh. He couldn't remember.

He glanced briefly at the two younger bikers sitting beside him.

Viper might have been covered in tattoos and carried himself like someone who'd seen more hardship than most people twice his age. Cullen had an easygoing nature that balanced Viper's dry humor surprisingly well but despite being younger than Drake, neither of them acted like it.

They looked after each other. Argued like brothers. Watched each other's backs without thinking about it. There was something refreshing about that. Something honest and since leaving the duplex, Drake didn't feel completely alone.

His thoughts drifted back to Ally. To Butterfly Academy. To the impossible mission he'd been turning over in his head for days.

He looked at Viper. Then Cullen.

Maybe he had stumbled across the first two people willing to stand beside him. The thought settled quietly in the back of his mind.

He wasn't ready to ask yet. They barely knew one another but hope, however small, flickered to life again.

For tonight, though, he pushed those thoughts aside. He leaned back against the headboard, took another sip of his beer, and laughed as Cullen loudly insisted the referee had missed an obvious foul.

For just a little while, the weight of Dragonfly Academy, Butterfly Academy, Helena, and Ally's uncertain fate faded into the background and Drake simply enjoyed having company.

Chapter Eighteen

The following morning, Drake was pulled from one of the deepest sleeps he could remember by the unmistakable sound of someone yelling.

"What the hell?!" A loud bang echoed through the motel wall. "Are you two out of your damn minds?!"

The shouting was immediately followed by hysterical laughter. Not just ordinary laughter. The kind that left people gasping for air.

Drake's eyes slowly opened. For a moment he simply stared at the stained motel ceiling, disoriented. He blinked a few times, trying to remember where he was.

The motel. Meeting Viper and Cullen. The boxing match. Beer.

He frowned.

"I actually fell asleep..." That realization alone was surprising. He couldn't even remember closing his eyes.

Normally sleep came in restless stretches, broken every hour or two by nightmares or memories he couldn't outrun.

Last night...nothing. He had simply drifted off. He carefully pushed himself upright. The movement tugged at his side.

He paused, expecting the familiar sharp pain from his wound. Instead, just a dull ache. Curious, he carefully lifted the edge of the fresh bandage.

The stitches held firmly. Not a single one had pulled loose.

"Huh..." He couldn't help smirking. "I'll be damned." He had honestly expected Cullen's improvised sewing job to come apart before morning but it seemed sturdier than the stitches the hospital had put in.

"They actually did a better job." Another shout came through the wall.

"You idiots!"

More laughter followed. Drake rubbed a hand across his bald head.

"What the hell are they doing now?" He looked around the room. The television was still on, though muted. Several empty beer bottles sat neatly beside the trash can. The bed beside him was empty.

Viper and Cullen were nowhere to be seen. Then the motel room door burst open. Viper stumbled inside first, doubled over with laughter. Cullen followed close behind, laughing so hard tears streamed down his face.

Neither one could seem to catch his breath. Behind them came another muffled yell from next door.

"I swear I'm gonna kill both of you!" The threat only made the pair laugh even harder.

Drake raised an eyebrow.

"What happened?" Neither answered immediately. They simply leaned against the wall, trying unsuccessfully to compose themselves.

Only then did Drake notice what Viper was carrying. An empty motel ice bucket. There was no plastic liner inside. No ice. Just a few lingering drops of water clinging to the bottom.

Drake slowly looked from the bucket to the two grinning bikers and then toward the wall separating their room from Hudson's.

Realization dawned.

"You two didn't..."

Viper couldn't even speak. Still laughing, he simply nodded.

Cullen finally managed to inhale enough air to explain.

"We dumped..." He burst into another fit of laughter. “A whole bucket..." Another laugh interrupted him. “Of ice water..." He pointed toward Hudson's room. "On Hudson while he was asleep."

Silence. Then another furious yell exploded through the wall.

"You two are dead!"

Viper nearly collapsed onto the bed laughing. Cullen had to grab the dresser to keep from falling over. Drake stared at them for several seconds. Then, despite himself...he laughed.

A genuine, helpless laugh escaped him.

"You idiots."

"Worth it," Viper wheezed. "So worth it."

"He deserved it."

Drake shook his head. Another muffled voice came from next door.

"I'm serious! I'll shave your heads while you sleep!"

Viper immediately shouted back through the wall.

"Too late for Drake!"

Cullen lost all composure again. Drake buried his face in one hand.

"You two have a death wish."

"We're already dead." Viper grinned. "We're just waiting for Hudson to collect."

Another pillow hit the shared wall from the opposite room. The dull thud made all three laugh again. Eventually the laughter faded.

The room settled into comfortable silence. Viper looked over at Drake.

"You hungry?"

Drake hadn't really thought about food. Then, as if on cue, his stomach let out a loud, unmistakable growl. All three men looked at it.

Cullen grinned.

"I'll take that as a yes."

Drake chuckled.

"I guess I haven't eaten much lately."

"Free breakfast." Viper nodded toward the motel office. "Lobby and it's actually hot."

Drake looked skeptical.

"It's motel food."

"I know but trust me, they've got eggs, bacon, sausage."

"Biscuits and gravy." Cullen added. "And waffles."

Drake raised an eyebrow.

"You're kidding."

"I wish."

"Cullen's already had two plates." Cullen didn't even try denying it.

"I'm considering a third."

Drake laughed.

"I don't know where you put it."

"Years of practice."

"Get dressed." Viper pointed toward Drake's backpack. "Breakfast ends in half an hour."

"We don't need Hudson eating everything before we get there."

A muffled voice immediately came through the wall.

"I heard that!"

Viper smirked.

"Good."

Drake climbed carefully off the bed. His side still ached, but it was manageable. He dug through his backpack until he found a clean shirt and another pair of jeans. As he changed clothes, he caught himself smiling. It felt... strange.

Only two days ago he'd been riding alone with no destination, convinced that the impossible task ahead of him would have to be faced by himself. Now...He'd somehow ended up sharing jokes with three wandering bikers he'd met completely by chance.

He wasn't foolish enough to think he truly knew them yet but he liked them. They were rough around the edges. Immature at times. Loud and annoying but underneath all of that...they looked after one another.

Even their prank on Hudson had the unmistakable feel of brothers teasing one another rather than men who genuinely wished each other harm. It stirred something inside Drake that he hadn't felt in years. A sense of belonging.

He wasn't ready to admit it aloud. Not even to himself but as he slung his jacket over one shoulder and followed Viper and Cullen toward the motel lobby, he realized this was the first morning in nearly a decade that he hadn't woken up feeling completely alone.

Drake hadn't realized how empty his stomach was until he walked into the motel lobby and caught the smell of breakfast.

Fresh bacon. Scrambled eggs. Sausage. Biscuits covered in peppered gravy. Toast popping from a conveyor toaster and waffles cooking in an iron near the end of the buffet.

His stomach growled loudly enough that Cullen looked over with a grin.

"Told you."

Drake couldn't argue with that. He grabbed one of the large white plates and began loading it. A scoop of scrambled eggs. Three sausage links. Several strips of bacon. A biscuit smothered in gravy.

He hesitated for only a second before adding another biscuit. By the time he reached the end of the buffet, the plate was stacked so high it looked like it might collapse.

"You planning on feeding the whole motel?" Cullen asked.

Drake glanced down at the mountain of food.

"I guess I was hungrier than I thought."

The three of them found an empty table near the window.

Morning sunlight streamed through the glass, warming the small dining area. Drake sat down and immediately picked up his fork.

Across from him, Viper had a single biscuit on his plate. Next to Drake, Cullen was enthusiastically working his way through what appeared to be his third plate of food that morning.

Drake looked between them. Then back to Cullen.

"You've already eaten all that?"

Cullen shrugged as if it were completely normal.

"I've got a fast metabolism."

"You've got a hollow leg," Viper muttered.

Cullen ignored him.

Drake finally looked at Viper.

"You're not hungry?"

Viper tore off a small piece of biscuit.

"I had a waffle earlier."

"Just one?"

"And some coffee."

Drake frowned.

"That's it?"

Viper nodded.

"I can't eat a lot." He shrugged casually. "If I do I usually end up getting sick."

Drake accepted the answer with a nod. Everyone's body worked differently. He stabbed a forkful of eggs and sausage.

The first bite nearly made him close his eyes. He hadn't had a hot breakfast in... he honestly couldn't remember how long. Most mornings on the road consisted of stale pastries, beef jerky, or whatever he happened to grab from a convenience store.

This felt like a feast. He quickly chased it with a long drink of orange juice. The cold citrus tasted just as good. Before he could take another bite, a chair scraped across the floor.

Hudson dropped into the seat across from him. His flame-red hair stuck up in several directions. He looked exhausted. His blue eyes narrowed immediately.

Drake couldn't help himself.

"You must be Princess Icy Pop."

For one long second, Hudson simply stared at him. Then Cullen snorted. Viper burst out laughing. Cullen quickly followed.

Hudson pointed accusingly at the pair.

"You told him."

"We absolutely did," Viper admitted proudly.

Hudson sighed dramatically.

"I hate both of you."

"This," Cullen said between chuckles, "is Hudson."

Hudson folded his arms.

"And who are you?" His eyes slowly swept over Drake's broad shoulders, bald head, and rugged face. "The Rock's ugly white cousin?"

For a split second there was complete silence. Then Viper nearly choked laughing. Cullen slapped the table. Even Drake couldn't stop himself.

"That's actually not bad," he admitted.

Viper wiped tears from his eyes.

"This is Drake." He pointed toward Drake's side. "Cullen stitched him up last night."

Hudson looked at the bandaged wound but didn't say anything.

"Long story." Drake said and Hudson nodded once. He went over poured himself a cup of coffee.

Cullen leaned toward Drake.

"Hudson isn't much of a morning person, especially after..." He glanced toward Hudson with a grin. "A long night."

Hudson rolled his eyes.

"Speaking of..." He looked around. "What happened to Sally?"

Viper shrugged.

"No idea, guessing she took her walk of shame before sunrise."

Cullen nodded. Hudson sighed.

"She also stole my wallet."

Silence. Then all three men laughed at once. Drake nearly spilled his orange juice.

"You serious?"

Hudson pulled his pockets inside out.

"I had almost two hundred bucks in there."

Viper laughed harder.

"I told you not to trust bar girls."

"She seemed trustworthy." Hudson grumbled.

"That was your first mistake." Cullen pointed his fork toward Hudson. "And it serves you right."

Hudson glared at him.

"You're all terrible friends."

"We're excellent friends." Viper corrected. "We're just not sympathetic."

Drake chuckled.

"It's the price we pay for taking strangers back to motel rooms."

Hudson looked at him hopefully.

"So you're on my side?"

Drake shook his head.

"Nope."

Hudson groaned.

"I learned a long time ago." Drake took another bite of eggs before continuing. "I don't keep anything important where someone else can get to it, my cash stays hidden and my important stuff stays with my bike so if somebody steals my wallet..." He shrugged. "They're getting maybe twenty bucks."

Hudson scowled.

"Would've been nice to know yesterday."

Viper smirked.

"Maybe next time don't think with the wrong head."

Cullen laughed loud enough to turn a few heads around the breakfast room. Hudson simply buried his face in his coffee mug.

"I hate all of you."

"No you don't." Viper nudged him with an elbow. "You'd miss us."

"Probably…" Hudson admitted quietly.

The table settled into comfortable conversation while everyone finished eating. Drake couldn't remember the last time breakfast had been this enjoyable. There was no tension. No suspicion.

Just four men teasing one another over cheap motel food. It felt... normal. Something he'd almost forgotten existed. As the plates gradually emptied, Viper glanced toward the parking lot through the window.

"We should probably get moving."

Drake looked up.

"You guys heading out already?"

Viper nodded.

"We don't usually stay in one place long."

Drake felt a flicker of disappointment. He hadn't known them very long. Barely a day yet he'd genuinely enjoyed their company.

Before he could think too much about it, Viper spoke again.

"You could always ride with us."

Drake blinked.

"If you're feeling up to it."

He instinctively rested a hand against the bandage beneath his shirt. The stitches barely hurt anymore. Certainly not enough to keep him off his motorcycle. More importantly...he didn't want to be alone again.

There was also something else. He wanted to know these three better. He wasn't about to ask strangers to help him take down the Academies. But maybe given enough time…they wouldn't be strangers anymore.

A small smile crossed his face.

"Sure." He nodded. "These stitches seem to be holding better than expected."

Cullen practically beamed.

"I should've been a doctor."

Viper laughed.

"You nearly passed out buying peroxide."

"I was overwhelmed."

"You got distracted by the candy aisle."

"There were gummy worms."

Hudson shook his head.

"I ride with children."

"We're charming."

"You're idiots."

"Both can be true."

Viper stood, gathering the empty plates. "Alright." He looked around the table. "We roll out in thirty minutes."

Everyone nodded.

Hudson continued sipping his coffee with the expression of a man still mourning both his stolen wallet and his dignity. Drake leaned back in his chair, surprisingly content.

The road ahead didn't seem quite so lonely and somewhere deep in the back of his mind, the impossible mission waiting for him no longer felt like something he had to face by himself.

Chapter Nineteen

The day passed more slowly than Drake thought they would.

Not because it was boring. Quite the opposite. Traveling with the Stray Sons made the endless highways feel shorter than they ever had before.

They rode together the entire day, the rumble of four motorcycles echoing across open stretches of road. When they stopped for fuel, one of them inevitably wandered into a convenience store while another checked over the bikes.

Hudson never seemed to lose his talent for getting himself into ridiculous situations.

At one of their meal stops, he managed to spill an entire cup of coffee into one of his saddlebags because he insisted he could ride while holding it.

That same evening he flirted with a waitress so enthusiastically that she accidentally dumped an entire basket of onion rings into his lap.

Viper and Cullen had laughed until they could barely breathe. Drake had laughed too. It surprised him how easily the laughter came now.

The three younger bikers bickered constantly. Hudson complained. Cullen teased him. Viper usually ended up playing referee while making sarcastic comments that somehow annoyed both of them equally.

They argued loudly. Insulted one another without mercy. Yet if anyone outside their little group so much as looked at one of them the wrong way, the other two were immediately at their side.

It was loyalty. The kind Drake hadn't experienced in a very long time but no matter how much he enjoyed their company...

His thoughts always found their way back to Ally.

Every single day.

He wondered where she slept. Whether she cried herself to sleep. Whether she was frightened. Whether she'd already begun believing the lies that were undoubtedly being fed to her.

Butterfly Academy didn't just hurt children. It reshaped them. Broke them. Then rebuilt them into whatever it wanted them to become.

Drake knew exactly how effective that process could be. He'd lived it himself and the longer Ally remained there...the harder it would be to undo the damage.

His chest tightened every time he thought about it. He couldn't keep putting this conversation off. Late that afternoon the group pulled into a lonely roadside rest area.

There wasn't much there. A few picnic tables. A pair of trash cans overflowing with fast-food wrappers. An old wooden information board missing half its maps.

No restroom.

Hudson sighed dramatically as he climbed off his motorcycle.

"Seriously?"

"Guess we're watering the trees again," Cullen said.

The four men wandered off in different directions to find a little privacy among the brush. Drake took care of business quickly before returning to the motorcycles.

He leaned against his Harley and rubbed the back of his neck. His stomach twisted with nerves. This was it. Either they thought he'd lost his mind Or...his thoughts were interrupted as Viper emerged from behind a cluster of trees, zipping up his jeans.

"The other two disappeared." Drake glanced toward the road. "They'll probably come back with snacks."

Viper nodded.

"I wasn't ready to get back on the bike yet."

Neither was Drake. The silence stretched between them. The evening sun had already begun sinking toward the horizon. Orange light reflected off chrome and windshields.

"Getting late," Drake finally said.

"Yeah." Viper leaned against his own motorcycle. "We'll need to figure out where we're sleeping."

Drake looked around.

"There anything nearby?"

"No idea." Viper shrugged. "If we've got enough cash we'll grab a motel."

"And if not?"

Viper smiled faintly.

"Sleeping bags." He pointed toward his saddlebags. "We all carry one, some nights that's all we've got."

Drake nodded slowly.

"Right."

He rubbed the back of his neck again. Viper watched him for a long moment.

"Something's bothering you."

It wasn't a question. Drake looked down at the gravel beneath his boots.

"Yeah..." He drew in a slow breath. "I've been wanting to ask you something."

Viper's expression became more serious.

"What is it?"

Drake hesitated. He'd spent days trying to figure out how to explain it. Nothing sounded sane.

"It's..." He sighed. "It's going to sound completely insane."

Viper folded his arms.

"Try me."

Drake stared out toward the empty highway.

"I grew up in a place called Dragonfly Academy."

Viper stayed silent.

"It looked like a boarding school." He swallowed hard. "But it wasn't, they didn't teach math or history, they taught fear."

He stopped there. The memories tried forcing themselves to the surface. He pushed them back down.

"I don't really want to get into everything that happened there."

Viper nodded once.

"You don't have to."

Drake appreciated that.

"My friend..." He corrected himself. "The closest thing I've got to a friend...has a nine-year-old daughter named Ally." His voice softened as he said her name. "A woman named Helena took her and her brother runs another place called Butterfly Academy."

Viper frowned.

"Same kind of place?"

"Yeah." Drake answered immediately. "They're connected, I couldn't stop them." He looked down at the scar beneath the fresh bandage on his side. "I tried but they sent some of the men I grew up with after me." He tapped the healing wound. "This is from them."

Viper's eyes narrowed.

"So that's how you got stabbed."

Drake nodded.

"They were sending me a message, to stay away but I can't." Silence settled between them. "I have to get Ally out." His jaw tightened. "But..." He looked directly at Viper. "I can't just rescue her, if I leave the others behind I'd be no better than the people who abandoned us."

His voice grew firmer.

"I want every kid out, I want both Academies shut down and I want Helena and everyone helping her behind bars."

Viper stared at him.

"You want our help."

Drake laughed bitterly.

"I know, it sounds ridiculous."

"It is ridiculous, there are only four of us and the people running these places have money, connections, even people inside law enforcement so I don't know who's safe to trust anymore."

He shook his head.

"I can't go to the police because I don't know who's already been bought but I can't do it alone so..." He took a breath. "I'm asking if you'll help me."

Viper looked thoughtfully toward the highway.

"So..." He spoke slowly. "You want four bikers to march into two heavily protected schools to rescue every child and somehow expose the people running them."

Drake rubbed the back of his neck again.

"When you say it like that…it sounds even crazier."

"It does."

Drake sighed.

"I know and I'd understand if you said no, I've only known you guys a few days I just..." His voice caught. "I can't leave Ally there and I couldn't live with myself if I only saved her."

The words hung heavily in the evening air. Viper studied him carefully. Not judging. Simply thinking.

"Alright."

Drake blinked.

"What?"

"We'll help."

Drake searched his face.

"You mean that?"

Viper nodded.

"When Hudson and Cullen get back we'll sit down, we'll hear everything and we'll figure out a plan."

Drake stared at him in disbelief.

"Just like that?"

Viper smiled.

"You've been riding with us."

"So?"

"So..." Viper shrugged as though it were obvious. "You're one of us now."

The words hit Drake harder than he'd expected. One of us. It had been years since anyone had made him feel like he belonged anywhere. His shoulders relaxed for what felt like the first time since Ally had been taken.

A slow breath escaped him.

"Thank you."

Viper clapped him once on the shoulder.

"No need." He grinned. "Besides, if these Academy people are half as awful as you say they're about overdue for someone to knock on their front door."

Drake laughed quietly. It was still dangerous. Still uncertain but now there was finally real hope for Ally.

Drake wasn't sure what woke him first.

The screech of tires or the shouting. His eyes snapped open.

For one confused moment, all he saw was the gray morning sky above the trees. Then another voice rang out, sharp and commanding, speaking a language he couldn't understand.

His brow furrowed.

"What?..."

He slowly pushed himself upright, immediately regretting it. A dull ache spread across his back. Sleeping directly on the hard ground had done him no favors. He reached behind himself and rubbed the sore muscles with a groan.

"Next stop..." He stretched carefully. "I'm getting us a motel. His voice was still thick with sleep. "I don't care if I have to pay for the whole damn thing."

Before anyone answered, he felt someone tap his arm. Cullen. The younger biker was already awake, crouched beside his rolled-up sleeping bag. He immediately pressed a finger against his lips.

"Shhh."

Drake frowned.

"What?"

Cullen silently pointed toward the other end of the rest area. Only then did Drake notice the commotion. A black SUV sat sideways across part of the parking lot, its windows tinted so dark they were almost mirror-like.

Three sharply dressed men stood outside it. All three wore expensive black suits despite the early morning heat. Two had pistols drawn, though they weren't pointing them at anyone. The third stood with his back perfectly straight beneath a charcoal fedora.

For a brief second Drake honestly wondered if he was still asleep.

"What..." He blinked several times. "The hell?..."

The whole scene looked like something out of an old gangster movie. The expensive SUV. The tailored suits. The polished dress shoes. Even the fedora.

It was so out of place beside a rundown roadside rest stop that it almost seemed ridiculous. Then he noticed who was standing opposite them.

Viper.

His arms were folded tightly across his chest. Even from where Drake sat, he could see the irritation written across his face. The man in the fedora said something in rapid Italian. Viper answered back in English just as sharply.

Drake looked between them.

"What in hell is going on?"

Hudson immediately leaned toward him.

"Keep your voice down."

Drake looked at him.

"You don't want them noticing us."

Drake glanced back toward the confrontation. Cullen quietly spoke one word.

"Roche."

Drake looked at him blankly.

"What?"

Cullen didn't elaborate. His attention remained fixed on Viper. The conversation continued. The fedora-wearing man remained remarkably calm.

Viper...Not so much. His gestures became more animated. At one point he threw both hands into the air in obvious frustration.

The older man answered in Italian again. His tone remained measured. That somehow seemed to irritate Viper even more.

Drake wished he understood a single word they were saying.

Finally, the man adjusted the brim of his fedora. He gave Viper one last look before speaking another short sentence in Italian. The two armed men holstered their pistols. All three climbed back into the SUV.

A second later the engine roared to life. The vehicle turned smoothly back onto the highway. As it disappeared around the bend, Viper raised both hands into the air. He flipped the departing SUV off with both middle fingers.

"Yeah!" He shouted after them. "Keep driving!"

The SUV never slowed. Within seconds it vanished completely. Silence settled over the rest area again.

Drake looked back toward Hudson and Cullen. Neither seemed particularly surprised. Instead, both simply began rolling up their sleeping bags as though this sort of thing happened every week.

Viper stalked back toward the campsite, muttering under his breath.

"I swear..." He yanked his sleeping bag off the ground. "He's got a damn tracker on me."

Drake stood.

"Who was that?"

Viper didn't even look up.

"No one you need to worry about." He stuffed the sleeping bag into its sack with considerably more force than necessary. "Come on, let's get moving."

Drake folded his arms.

"No."

Viper stopped.

"I said let's—"

"Not until you tell me what in the hell that was."

The campsite grew quiet. Hudson exchanged a quick glance with Cullen. Viper stared at Drake for several long seconds.

Then sighed heavily.

"Fine…" He rubbed his forehead. "That was Levon Roche."

Drake waited. Nothing.

"Okay?"

Viper blinked.

"Head of Roche Pride."

Drake tilted his head.

"I still don't know what that means."

Now Viper looked genuinely confused.

"The mafia."

Silence.

"You've seriously never heard of Roche Pride?"

Drake shrugged.

"I mean…maybe I've heard the name before but I never paid attention." He scratched the back of his neck. "I honestly thought if I ever met a mafia boss..." He gestured toward the road. "He wouldn't actually look like he walked straight out of a gangster movie."

Hudson snorted. Cullen burst into laughter. Even Viper looked like he was trying not to smile but then he shot both of them an annoyed glare.

"Don't encourage him."

That only made Hudson laugh harder. Drake looked between the three of them.

"So..." He pointed toward the highway. "Why was an actual mafia boss looking for you?"

Viper immediately became serious again.

"I don't have time to explain."

"Why not?"

"Because..." He slung his pack over one shoulder. "If I keep thinking about that conversation, "I'm going to lose what's left of my fucking patience."

Drake could tell from his expression that the subject was closed. At least for now. Whatever history existed between Viper and Levon Roche clearly wasn't something he wanted to discuss out in the open.

Drake decided not to push. Not yet. Instead he began cleaning up their little campsite. Empty soda cans. Burger wrappers. Paper napkins blowing in the breeze.

He gathered everything into one armful and carried it to the nearby overflowing trash bin. Someone had balanced coffee cups and fast-food bags on top of the pile, and several wrappers had blown onto the ground around it.

Drake shoved their trash as far inside as he could before brushing his hands together. When he turned around, Hudson was already strapping his sleeping bag to his motorcycle.

Cullen was checking the tension on one of his saddlebags. Viper stood silently beside his own bike, still wearing the same irritated expression. Drake couldn't stop wondering about the strange encounter.

An actual mafia boss. Speaking fluent Italian. Showing up at a lonely roadside rest stop just to confront Viper. None of it made any sense and judging by the way Hudson and Cullen had reacted, it wasn't the first time.

He walked back to his Harley, tightened the straps holding his backpack in place, and swung one leg over the seat. The familiar weight of the handlebars settled into his hands. He started the engine but didn't pull away.

He waited patiently while the others finished packing. Whatever secrets Viper was keeping, Drake had a feeling they would eventually come to light and somehow, he suspected those secrets

were far bigger than a chance encounter with a man named Levon Roche.

Chapter Twenty

Drake insisted they stop at the very next motel they came across. He wasn't sleeping on the ground again. Not after waking up feeling like someone had taken a sledgehammer to his back.

"I don't care if I have to pay for the room myself," he'd grumbled as they rode. "I'm too old for that camping shit."

Hudson had laughed loud enough for it to be heard over the rumble of the motorcycles.

"You've slept on worse."

"I have," Drake admitted. "Doesn't mean I'm doing it again."

Even Viper had managed the faintest hint of a smile despite his foul mood. The encounter with Levon Roche had lingered over the group like a storm cloud for the rest of the day.

Viper barely spoke.

Normally he was the one who kept Hudson and Cullen from arguing themselves into circles, but now he simply rode in silence with his eyes fixed on the highway.

No sarcastic remarks. No teasing. Nothing.

Hudson and Cullen didn't try to get him talking. They clearly knew better. Whatever had happened between Viper and Levon wasn't something either of them wanted to poke at.

Drake took his cue from them. He had questions. Far too many of them but he kept every single one to himself.

Late that afternoon they found a modest roadside motel. It wasn't anything special. The faded vacancy sign buzzed loudly. Several letters no longer lit up. The paint peeled from the railings outside the second-floor rooms, and the office smelled faintly of stale coffee and old carpet.

Drake paid for a room with two queen beds. The four of them had crowded into it without complaint. Hudson immediately claimed one side of a bed while Cullen sprawled across the other.

Viper had simply kicked off his boots and collapsed without saying much of anything. Drake had taken the remaining space.

Compared to sleeping on hard-packed dirt, the mattress felt like heaven.

The next morning, Drake woke with a long yawn. He stretched until several joints popped loudly.

"Mmm..." He rolled his shoulders. His back still ached, but nowhere near as badly as it had after sleeping outside. "Much better..." he muttered.

He sat up slowly and rubbed the sleep from his tired green eyes. Morning sunlight spilled through the gap in the curtains.

The room was quiet. Drake frowned.

"Guys?"

No answer. He swung his legs over the edge of the bed. The other mattress was empty. Blankets tossed aside.

No Hudson. No Cullen. No Viper.

He assumed they'd gone to grab breakfast. Still half asleep, he pulled on his ripped jeans and tank top before shoving his feet into his boots.

As he reached for his backpack, something caught his eye. A folded piece of paper sat on top of the dresser. The television remote rested on it to keep it from blowing away beneath the air conditioner.

Drake walked over. His stomach tightened. He picked it up and unfolded it. The handwriting was unmistakably Viper's.

Drake,

I'm sorry, but this is where we go our separate ways. I know I said we would help you with that rescue mission, but my life is way too messy right now and I don't want to get you caught up in all the bullshit with Levon. I meant what I said when I said you're one of us, and if we ever cross paths again, you'll be welcome wherever I am.

I wish you the best, and I hope you're able to rescue that little girl.

Stay cool.

Viper

Drake read it again. Then a third time. His jaw clenched tighter with every word.

"...Son of a bitch." The paper crumpled loudly inside his fist. He hurled it across the room. It bounced off the trash can before falling inside.

Silence returned. Drake stared at it. They were gone. All three of them. No goodbye. No handshake. No waking him up before they left. Just...a note.

He let out a bitter laugh.

"So much for being one of us."

The words echoed around the empty room. His chest tightened. He hated it. Not because they had left. Because for a few short days he'd allowed himself to believe he'd finally found people he could trust. People who hadn't looked at him like he was broken. People who laughed with him.

Argued with him. Shared motel rooms with him. People who had actually listened when he talked about Ally. He hadn't felt alone but now the silence in the motel room reminded him exactly what his life had always been.

Temporary. Everyone left eventually. A tear escaped before he could stop it. It slid slowly down his rough cheek.

"Damn it..." He angrily wiped it away with the heel of his hand. He wasn't crying over them. He told himself that. He was crying because with them gone so was his plan.

Four men had barely been enough to imagine taking on the Academies. One man? It wasn't possible. Not against Helena and Harold and not against everyone protecting them.

His thoughts drifted to Ally. Nine years old. Scared. Confused. Locked inside Butterfly Academy. He shut his eyes.

"I'll come back for you." His voice was barely above a whisper. "I swear I will." He rested both hands on the dresser. "Just..." He swallowed hard. "Please let Harold have enough compassion not to force you into anything you're not ready for."

He hated himself for even thinking it. Harold wasn't compassionate. None of them were. Still it was the only hope he had left. He wasn't going to save her today or tomorrow. Maybe not even this year.

The realization settled heavily onto his shoulders. His dream had simply been too big. Too ambitious. He'd expected three strangers he'd known less than a week to risk their lives for children they'd never met.

Looking back, he couldn't really blame them for walking away. Levon Roche was obviously a problem of their own. Whatever history

Viper had with that mafia boss was clearly serious enough that he'd chosen to disappear rather than drag Drake into it.

It still hurt but Drake understood. He picked up his backpack and slung it over one shoulder. There wasn't any reason to stay.

He walked to the door, opened it, and slammed it hard enough that the windows rattled.

"So much for the Stray Sons." He stalked across the parking lot without looking back. "They obviously didn't give a shit."

The words came out harsher than he truly meant. Deep down he knew Viper hadn't left because he didn't care. He'd left because he did.

That somehow made it sting even more. Drake reached his Harley and strapped on his backpack. As he tightened the buckle, another thought slowly formed. If three young bikers trying to survive on the road couldn't help him then maybe he was looking in the wrong place.

He didn't need three drifters. He needed an army. His gaze drifted toward the endless highway stretching beyond the motel.

"A real motorcycle club..." he muttered. "One with numbers, resources, and people who aren't afraid of getting their hands dirty."

He climbed onto the Harley. The engine roared to life beneath him. His destination was still unknown but now at least he had a direction.

Somewhere out there, there had to be a club big enough, strong enough, and crazy enough to help him bring the Academies crashing down once and for all.

Chapter Twenty-One

Several days passed before Drake finally found himself pulling into a city he had never seen before.

Except this time he wasn't just wandering. He needed to find a motorcycle club. Not just any club either. He needed men who understood loyalty. Men who weren't afraid of getting their hands dirty. Men who wouldn't back down when things became dangerous because what he was planning wasn't some simple rescue mission.

The last few nights had been spent drifting from bar to bar, listening carefully whenever bikers walked through the doors.

He watched patches. Listened to conversations. Studied the way they carried themselves.

Some clubs were nothing more than groups of guys looking for an excuse to drink and fight. Others were too small, too disorganized, or too wrapped up in their own problems.

None of them felt right. None of them felt like the kind of people he could trust with something this important and after several nights of searching...he was exhausted.

He needed sleep. He was riding through the unfamiliar city, scanning the roads for a vacancy sign, when something caught his attention.

A flickering neon glow reflected against the pavement. The sign was old but bright. Then he heard it. Motorcycle engines. Multiple engines. The deep rumble rolled through the streets.

Drake slowed. He turned his head toward the sound. A group of bikes. A lot of them. Curiosity got the better of him. He followed the sound down a side road until he found himself pulling into the parking lot of what was clearly not just a random hangout.

This was a clubhouse.

A real one. The building was large, reinforced, and surrounded by motorcycles. The sign hanging above the entrance flickered in bright red letters.

IRON REQUIEM

Drake stared at it for a moment. Now this looked promising. He pulled his Harley into the lot and stopped. For a moment, he simply sat there.

The place had a presence. A reputation. He could feel it. He didn't notice the way conversations had stopped. He didn't notice the footsteps approaching. He didn't notice the dozens of eyes watching him. Not until the silence became too heavy.

Slowly, Drake looked around. His hand rested casually on the handlebars. Around him stood several bikers.

Leather cuts. Tattoos. Hard expressions. Every single one of them looked like they were waiting for him to make the wrong move.

Drake raised his eyebrows.

"Hello." No one answered. He cleared his throat. "Hope I'm not interrupting anything."

Still nothing.

"I heard your bikes and I was curious." He looked around at the group. "I'm not looking for trouble."

The bikers didn't move.

Didn't relax. If anything, their silence made them more intimidating. Finally, one man stepped forward. He was tall, broad-shouldered, and wore an expression that suggested he wasn't interested in wasting time.

"This is Iron Requiem territory." His voice was flat. "And we don't take kindly to strangers showing up uninvited."

Drake slowly nodded. He looked around.

"I wasn't trying to disrespect anyone." He paused. "I was actually looking for a club." A few of the bikers exchanged glances. "A club to join," Drake clarified. The man in front of him gave a humorless laugh.

"You picked a strange way to introduce yourself."

Drake shrugged.

"I've never been very good at introductions."

Before the conversation could go any further, another voice cut through the tension.

"Macon."

The entire group shifted.

A man stepped forward from the crowd. Drake immediately noticed the difference. This man didn't need to raise his voice. Didn't need to threaten anyone.

Everyone simply moved aside for him. He had dark skin, a shaved head, and a thick beard with streaks of gray running through it.

His steel-blue eyes were sharp. Observant. The kind of eyes that missed nothing. The man looked toward Macon.

"What have I told you about being hostile to guests?"

Macon lowered his gaze slightly.

"Sorry, Grim." He motioned toward Drake. "Was just giving him a warning."

The man gave him a look.

Macon immediately stepped back. Drake filed that away. This man commanded respect. Not demanded it. Earned it.

He turned his attention back to him. "Darius Crowe." He introduced himself. "People call me Grim." He glanced toward the clubhouse. "I own this club." Then his eyes narrowed slightly. "And you are?"

"Drake." He held out his hand. Darius looked at it. For a moment, Drake thought he might accept. He didn't. The older man simply looked back at him.

"And you want to join my club?"

Drake lowered his hand.

"I might."

That earned a slight reaction. Darius tilted his head.

"Most men come in here begging for a place."

Drake shrugged.

"I'm not most men." A few bikers smirked. Drake continued. "But I'm tired of being a lone wolf." The words felt strange coming out of his mouth.

He had spent years convincing himself he didn't need anyone.

That being alone was safer but after meeting Viper, Cullen, and Hudson...After realizing what it felt like to have people beside him...He knew he couldn't keep doing everything alone.

"So yeah." He looked directly at Darius. "I'm looking for somewhere to belong."

Darius studied him.

"Do you know what you're asking for?"

Drake nodded.

"An MC."

"No." Darius stepped closer. "You're asking to become part of something bigger than yourself, you're asking to be responsible for people who will expect you to stand beside them, you're asking to put your life in the hands of men who will expect you to do the same."

Drake didn't hesitate.

"I know."

Darius stared at him.

"And you still want it?"

"Yes." The answer came immediately. Darius was quiet for several seconds.

"Possibly."

Drake raised an eyebrow.

"Possibly?"

"You don't just walk into Iron Requiem and become one of us." Darius looked him over. "You prove yourself."

Drake crossed his arms.

"How?"

A slow grin formed on Darius' face.

"That depends."

"On what?

"On whether you're actually as tough as you think you are."

Drake almost smiled.

"I can handle myself."

Darius' grin widened.

"Everyone says that." He turned slightly toward the clubhouse. "Most of them learn otherwise."

Drake stared at him. The challenge was obvious and maybe that was exactly what he needed. A test. A chance. A way to prove he wasn't just some angry man chasing an impossible dream.

"I'm up for it." The words came out confident. Certain. Darius looked at him for another moment. Then he chuckled. Not cruelly. Almost approvingly but something about that grin made Drake's instincts flare.

He had seen that expression before. Right before someone gave him a challenge that was going to hurt. A lot.

Drake slowly exhaled. Yeah. Maybe he had just bitten off more than he could chew but after everything he had survived...He wasn't about to back down now.

Darius looked Drake up and down for another long moment before motioning for him to follow.

"Bring your bike."

Drake swung a leg over his Harley and started the engine. One by one the members of Iron Requiem climbed onto their own motorcycles until the quiet parking lot was once again filled with the thunder of V-twin engines.

No one explained where they were going.

Drake didn't ask. If this was the beginning of whatever test Darius had in mind, he wasn't about to start by questioning orders.

The group rode through the city before leaving the pavement behind. The smooth highway gave way to cracked asphalt, then gravel, and finally an overgrown dirt road that wound through dense woods. Branches hung low over the trail, occasionally scraping against helmets and shoulders.

After nearly twenty minutes they arrived at what looked like an abandoned logging site. Rusted machinery sat half-swallowed by weeds. Rotten stacks of timber leaned dangerously against one another. An old water tower stood crooked in the distance.

The bikers parked in a loose semicircle. Darius climbed off his motorcycle and folded his arms.

"This place belongs to us."

Drake looked around.

"It doesn't look like much."

"It isn't supposed to." A few of the members chuckled. Darius ignored them. "You said you're tired of being a lone wolf."

"I am."

"You said you're willing to do whatever it takes."

"I meant it."

Darius nodded once.

"Good."

He pointed toward a massive pile of old railroad ties that had collapsed beside one of the buildings.

"See those?"

Drake nodded.

"They need to be moved into the shed before morning."

Drake frowned.

"That's it?"

Macon laughed.

"You'll wish it was just that."

Darius continued.

"Some weigh close to two hundred pounds, they're soaked, they're splintered, and the ground is uneven. He pointed toward an old utility building nearly a hundred yards away. "You'll move every single one."

"By myself?"

"Yes."

Drake looked at the enormous pile. There had to be at least forty of them.

Darius wasn't finished.

"When you're done..." He pointed farther into the property. "There's an old generator, it hasn't worked in years, fix it." He shrugged. "If you can't, you fail."

Drake glanced between the pile and the distant shed.

"When do I stop?"

"When everything is done. "No time limit. No breaks mentioned. Nothing. Drake rolled his shoulders.

"Alright."

Without another word he walked toward the pile. The first railroad tie nearly proved Darius wasn't exaggerating. Drake crouched, wrapped both arms around the weathered wood and lifted. Nothing. He adjusted his footing, grunted, and finally the heavy timber broke free from the mud with a loud sucking sound.

He staggered under its weight before settling it across one shoulder. His stitched wound immediately protested. Pain shot across his ribs. He gritted his teeth.

One step. Then another.

By the tenth tie sweat poured off him. By the twentieth his shoulders felt like they were on fire. Splinters covered his palms. His lower back screamed every time he bent over. The members of Iron Requiem watched from the shade, saying very little.

Some clearly expected him to quit. Others simply observed. Hours passed. The dim moonlight provided little to see by.

Drake stumbled more than once across loose rocks. Halfway through another load his boot slipped in the mud. The heavy timber shifted unexpectedly and he lost his balance. The railroad tie slammed into his shoulder before throwing him sideways. He crashed hard against a jagged rock.

A sharp pain exploded through his knee.

"Damn it!" He sucked in a breath.

Blood slowly trickled from a long scrape along his forearm. His knee throbbed. For several seconds he remained where he'd fallen.

Macon stepped forward.

"That's enough, he'll never finish."

Darius held up a hand.

"No."

They watched silently as Drake planted both hands beneath himself. His injured knee nearly buckled as he stood. He leaned heavily on the railroad tie for balance. His breathing was ragged.

Every instinct told him to stop. To admit defeat but he hoisted the timber back onto his shoulder anyway.

"I'm...not..." He took another step. "Finished."

Macon shook his head.

"Idiot."

One of the older members beside him smiled faintly.

"No, he just doesn't quit."

At last the final railroad tie slid into place inside the shed. Drake dropped to one knee, breathing so heavily he could barely see straight. His shirt clung to him with sweat.

Mud covered his jeans. His scraped arm had dried with streaks of blood running toward his wrist. Darius finally walked over.

"You done?"

Drake looked up.

"Barely."

"The generator."

Drake laughed once. It sounded more exhausted than amused.

"I figured you'd forgotten."

"I don't forget."

Drake slowly climbed back to his feet. Every muscle in his body protested. He limped toward the old generator sitting beside the maintenance building. He removed the rusted cover.

Immediately he saw years of neglect. Frayed wiring. Corroded battery terminals. A clogged fuel line. He worked methodically. Cleaning. Replacing wire with spare pieces scavenged from nearby equipment. Draining old fuel and adjusting connections.

His father had taught him enough before Dragonfly Academy stole him away. Those lessons had earned him jobs all over the country. Now they might earn him a place here.

Nearly another hour passed. The early morning sun settled over the property, but it was still overcast. The members gathered nearby. Drake wiped greasy hands on his jeans.

"Moment of truth." He reached for the starter. Nothing. Silence. He frowned and opened the panel again. Checked everything. Then spotted it. One loose ground wire.

He tightened it and closed the cover once more.

"Come on..." He pressed the starter again. The engine coughed. Backfired loudly. Several bikers stepped backward and then the old generator roared to life.

Lights mounted around the property flickered once...twice...then glowed steadily.

A cheer erupted from several members.

Macon folded his arms.

"I'll be damned."

Drake leaned against the generator, completely spent. Darius approached slowly.

"You got hurt."

Drake looked at the scrape on his arm.

"I've had worse."

"Your knee."

"It'll heal."

"You almost quit."

Drake met his eyes.

"No, I fell but I never thought about quitting."

Silence stretched between them.

Finally, Darius smiled. This time it wasn't the amused grin from earlier. It was one of genuine respect.

"Good answer."

He extended his hand and Drake took it. Darius's grip was firm.

"You passed." A grin slowly spread across Drake's tired face. "Welcome to Iron Requiem, Prospect."

The members around them nodded in approval. Some clapped him on the shoulder as they walked past. Even Macon stopped beside him.

"I honestly thought you'd quit after that fall." Drake smirked despite the pain. Macon laughed. "But you didn't."

"No." Drake looked around at the men gathered beneath the newly restored lights with pride. He felt as though he had finally found somewhere he might belong.

He still had a long road ahead before he could rescue Ally and destroy the Academies but now he wouldn't have to walk that road alone.

Chapter Twenty-Two

Drake drifted slowly toward consciousness.

At first, all he knew was warmth. Then pressure.

Firm hands worked their way across his back, pressing into muscles that felt like they had been tied into knots. He let out a long, involuntary groan as the tension slowly began to ease.

"Mm..."

His face was buried in a pillow that smelled faintly of laundry detergent and cigarette smoke.

For a brief moment he couldn't remember where he was. The last thing he clearly recalled was standing in front of the old generator at Iron Requiem's abandoned logging site.

He remembered tightening the last ground wire, hearing the engine roar to life, and seeing the lights flicker on around the property.

After that...nothing.

The hands dug into another tight muscle between his shoulder blades.

"Ah..."

Drake winced. Then another thought finally cut through the haze. Someone was touching him. His eyes snapped open. His body instinctively tensed.

"Who are..." He tried to roll over but immediately regretted it as pain shot through his shoulders and ribs. "Who are you?..."

The woman stopped massaging him and stepped back enough for him to see her clearly. She couldn't have been much younger than him. She had short brown hair that framed a friendly face, warm brown eyes, and bronze-colored skin. She wore jeans, a black tank top with an Iron Requiem patch stitched over the chest, and comfortable work boots.

She smiled softly.

"They call me Bunny."

Drake blinked.

"Bunny?"

She shrugged.

"Not the name my mama gave me, but it's the one everybody uses."

Drake slowly pushed himself into a sitting position. Every muscle protested, his back burned and his shoulders felt bruised. His knee still throbbed from where he'd fallen beneath the railroad tie.

"Hell..." He rubbed both hands over his face. "What happened?"

Bunny folded her arms.

"You've been out cold for a day and a half."

Drake stared at her.

"What?...a day and a half?"

She couldn't help giggling at the expression on his face.

"Darius came in here yesterday morning to check on you." She grinned. "You were sleeping so hard he thought you'd died."

Drake frowned.

"Seriously?"

"Mhmm, he stood there staring at you for almost a full minute." She mimicked Darius' deep voice. "Somebody poke him." She laughed. "When you still didn't move, Grim looked genuinely worried."

Drake rubbed the back of his neck.

"I guess I was more tired than I thought."

"You were beyond tired." Bunny sat on the edge of a nearby chair. "You pushed yourself way too hard." She pointed toward his scraped forearm. "We cleaned your cuts." She nodded toward his swollen knee." Wrapped that and Macon carried you in here after you passed out."

Drake raised an eyebrow.

"Macon? The same guy who thought I was going to quit?"

"The very same." She smiled. "He complained the whole way...this idiot weighs a ton."

Drake chuckled despite the soreness.

"I'll have to thank him."

"You probably should."

"He'd never admit it but he was worried too."

Drake slowly swung his legs over the side of the bed. The moment his feet touched the floor he hissed through clenched teeth.

"Damn..."

His entire body ached. The railroad ties had punished muscles he didn't even know existed. His knee pulsed with every heartbeat. His shoulders felt as though they had been beaten with baseball bats.

"I don't suppose..." He looked hopefully toward Bunny. "You have anything stronger than wishful thinking for the pain?"

She smiled knowingly.

"I figured you'd ask." Reaching over to the nightstand, she picked up a small prescription bottle and handed it to him. "Take a couple, they'll take the edge off."

Drake turned the bottle over in his hand. He didn't recognize the name on the label. He shrugged. At this point, he didn't particularly care what they were. If they helped him walk without feeling like he'd been run over by a truck, that was enough.

Bunny stood.

"Oh." She pointed toward the bathroom. "You might want to get cleaned up."

Drake looked down at himself. His clothes were filthy. Dried mud still clung to his jeans.

Grease from the generator stained his tank top. His arms were streaked with dried blood and dirt.

"Yeah, I probably smell about as good as I look."

Bunny laughed.

"Pretty close." She headed toward the door. "Darius wants to see you once you're up."

Drake nodded.

"I'll be there."

She paused with her hand on the doorknob.

"And Drake?" He looked up. "Welcome to Iron Requiem."

She offered him one last smile before disappearing into the hallway. The room fell quiet again.

Drake sat there for another moment. His gaze drifted to the pill bottle in his hand. He twisted the cap off and shook two small white tablets into his palm.

"Here's hoping..." he muttered.

A bottle of water sat beside the bed. He grabbed it, tossed the pills into his mouth, and swallowed them with several long drinks.

The cool water felt surprisingly refreshing. After setting the bottle aside, he leaned over and pulled his worn backpack closer.

The zipper rasped loudly as he opened it. He didn't have much in the way of clean clothes left. One clean pair of jeans, a handful of socks, and a spare tank top. He pulled them out and frowned.

"I'm running out."

He'd have to find a laundromat soon or buy more assuming prospects actually got paid around here. He wasn't even sure how Iron Requiem operated yet. As he carried the clothes toward the bathroom, his thoughts wandered.

Joining Iron Requiem...was it really the right decision? He still barely knew these people.

Darius had tested him harder than anyone had in years. Macon seemed like the type who enjoyed making prospects miserable. Bunny was friendly enough but he hadn't even learned all of their names and yet despite all of that...he couldn't deny the feeling settling quietly in the back of his mind.

It was better than being alone. After years of drifting from town to town with no destination and no one waiting for him...there was something strangely comforting about waking up somewhere people had bothered to take care of him.

Someone had cleaned his wounds. Someone had carried him to a bed. Someone had checked to make sure he was still breathing. It wasn't much but to Drake Rathburn, it felt like the closest thing to a home he'd had since he was twelve years old.

He quietly closed the bathroom door behind him and turned on the shower, hoping the hot water would wash away at least some of the aches that still clung stubbornly to his body.

Chapter Twenty-Three

Six months had passed since that rain-soaked night when everything changed, and now Drake found himself standing before the imposing wrought-iron gates of The Butterfly Academy, his boots planted firmly on the cobblestone path as though the simple act of standing still required enormous effort.

The building loomed before him like a gilded cage—Victorian architecture painted in deceptive pastels of cream and rose, with ivy crawling up its weathered stone façade like grasping fingers. Stained glass windows caught the afternoon light, casting fractured rainbows across the manicured lawn, but Drake knew better than to be fooled by the aesthetic charm. Behind those ornate walls, girls were kept like prized specimens, their autonomy stripped away under the guise of education and refinement.

The autumn wind whipped through the line of oak trees flanking the entrance, sending copper-colored leaves spiraling through the air. Drake shivered, though not from the cold. His leather jacket, worn at the elbows and smelling faintly of tobacco and motor oil, did little to insulate him from the chill that had settled deep in his bones—the kind of cold that came from anticipation and fear.

He wasn't alone. The presence of Darius Crowe at his right shoulder felt like an anchor, steadying him. The older man stood with his customary stillness, hands tucked into the pockets of his long charcoal coat, his silver-streaked beard catching the sunlight. Behind them, the Iron Requiem crew formed a loose semicircle—Macon with his massive arms crossed over his chest, scanning the perimeter with the alertness of a former soldier; Bunny leaning against her motorcycle, her brown eyes hidden behind mirrored sunglasses, chewing gum with rhythmic precision; and then Ruben Pierce and Cole Mercer, identical in their black tactical gear, standing so still they might have been statues.

Drake's fingers twitched at his sides, itching for the comfort of a cigarette, but he resisted. He needed his hands free. His heart hammered against his ribs in a staccato rhythm that seemed to count down toward something inevitable. Six months of searching of dead ends and whispered rumors in back-alley bars, of sleepless nights haunted by the thought of Ally's being taken her away. Six months, and here he was, finally facing the institution that had swallowed her whole.

The gates creaked open with a sound like an old man groaning, and Harold Lithen emerged. His reddish-brown hair was swept back with too much pomade, and his charcoal suit—clearly expensive, clearly tailored—hung on his frame with the precision of a man who cared deeply about appearances. He walked with the unhurried confidence of someone who believed he owned the ground he walked upon, which, in a very real sense, he did. The Butterfly Academy was his kingdom, and the girls within it his subjects.

"Drake," Harold called out, his voice carrying across the distance with practiced warmth that didn't reach his eyes. Those pale blue eyes, sharp and assessing, flickered over the assembled group, cataloging threats, calculating odds. "I must say, I'm surprised to see you here and with such...company."

Darius said nothing, merely inclining his head in the slightest of nods, his expression unreadable.

Drake stepped forward, his boots crunching against the gravel.

"I'm here about Ally," he said, and his voice came out rougher than intended, scraped raw by six months of silence on the subject. He cleared his throat, trying to steady himself. "I want her out of here. Now."

Harold's lips curved into a smile that held no humor.

"You know that's not how it works, Drake," Harold said. He took a step closer, close enough that Drake could see the years of guilt in his cobalt eyes. "Ally is and always was property of this academy. She was born here, you see. Her parents signed her over when she was three days old. Standard procedure for those who cannot afford to keep their children but recognize the value of our...educational opportunities." He paused, taking in a breath and exhaling before continuing. "We are her guardians now. Legally, morally, practically. She belongs here."

Drake closed his eyes, forcing himself to breathe. The words "belongs here" reverberated through his skull like a hammer strike. When he opened his eyes again, the world had taken on a sharper edge, hyper-real in its clarity—the individual leaves on the trees, the rust spot on Harold's lapel, the way Macon's jaw had tightened almost imperceptibly behind him.

"She had a life outside of this place, Harold," Drake said, his voice dropping to something dangerously quiet. He took another step forward, invading Harold's personal space, ignoring the way the older man's bodyguards—previously hidden in the shadows of the gatehouse—shifted into view. "She was thriving. She had friends, she was learning to play the guitar—badly, but she was learning. She laughed, Harold. I heard her laugh. She should never have been brought back here; torn away from everything she was building."

He could feel the heat rising in his chest, the familiar burn of helpless anger that had been his constant companion these past months.

"And if Donovan won't step up and take responsibility for her—if her own father is too much of a coward to face what he created—then I will. Let her come with me, and you'll never have to see either of us again. We'll disappear. You can pretend we never existed, that this little rebellion never happened."

Drake stared directly into Harold's deep blue eyes, refusing to blink, refusing to show weakness.

"I don't want to have to do this by force," he said, and the threat hung in the air between them, heavy as storm clouds. "But I will. I absolutely will."

For a long moment, the only sound was the wind in the trees and the distant chirping of birds. Harold studied him with the detached curiosity of a scientist observing a particularly interesting insect. Then he sighed, a sound of genuine disappointment, as though Drake were a student who had failed to grasp a simple lesson.

"We're not looking for a fight with you and your friends here, Drake," Harold said, his tone almost paternal, which made it somehow worse. "Truly, we're not. Violence is so...distasteful and bad for business. The Butterfly Academy has existed for so many years because we understand the value of discretion, of maintaining good relationships with the community but I will not be handing Ally or any of the other girls over to you. Not without proper compensation."

He smiled then, a shark's smile, all teeth and hunger. "And I know you don't have the money to be able to purchase a butterfly, Drake. A single butterfly—fully trained, fully educated, fully prepared for her role in society—carries a price tag of roughly five grand. That's the investment we've made in Ally's upbringing, her care, her training. Do you have five thousand dollars, Drake? Do your friends here have five thousand dollars?"

Drake felt the blood drain from his face. Five thousand. The number seemed absurd, impossible, a wall built specifically to keep people like him out. His hands curled into fists at his sides, his nails digging crescent moons into his palms. He opened his mouth to speak—to bargain, to beg, to threaten—but before he could form words, he felt Darius's hand settle on his shoulder.

The weight of that hand was firm, grounding, and immovable.

"Come on," Darius said, his voice low and steady, carrying the authority of someone who had commanded rooms far more dangerous than this. "We'll figure something out later."

"But, Grim—" Drake started, the nickname slipping out, his desperation cracking his voice. He couldn't just walk away. Not again.

Ally was in there, somewhere behind those walls, probably wondering if anyone was coming for her, if anyone cared—

"Come. Now." Darius's tone brooked no argument. His fingers tightened on Drake's shoulder, not painful but insistent, a signal that only Drake could interpret: Not here. Not now. Trust me.

Drake's throat felt tight, constricted by a tangle of rage and despair. He looked once more at Harold, memorizing the man's smug expression, storing it away for future reference. Then he looked at the academy itself, at the third-floor window where he knew Ally's room was—the corner room with the view of the garden. Was she looking out right now? Could she see him? Did she know he had tried?

He exhaled slowly, the breath shuddering out of him like a physical surrender. "Fine," he muttered, though the word tasted like ash. He turned, his boots scraping against the cobblestones, and began walking back toward where the motorcycles were parked along the curb.

As he passed Macon, he didn't see the almost imperceptible nod that Darius gave the large man—a slight dip of the chin, a flicker of the eyes toward the eastern wing of the building. Macon's expression didn't change, his arms remained crossed, but his stance shifted slightly, his weight moving to the balls of his feet, ready.

Drake didn't see the way Bunny's hand drifted toward her jacket pocket, fingers brushing against the shape of something metallic and important.

He didn't see the twins exchange a glance, silent communication passing between them, a plan already forming in the space between heartbeats.

All Drake saw was the pavement in front of him, blurring slightly at the edges, his vision swimming with the frustrated tears he refused to let fall. He walked away from The Butterfly Academy with his head held high and his heart in ruins, not knowing that the war had only just begun, and that surrender was merely the opening move in a game he didn't yet understand he was playing.

Drake spent the next several days in a restless haze, the kind of sleepless fog that settles into a man's bones and makes every hour feel stretched thin and brittle. He drifted through the cramped confines of Bunny's small camper in a state of perpetual agitation, unable to sit still for more than a few minutes at a time without feeling the need to move, to pace, to burn off the nervous energy that had been building inside him like steam in a sealed kettle. The camper's walls seemed to close in on him more with each passing day, the narrow galley kitchen and the fold-down table and the sleeping berth above the cab becoming a prison of its own making.

He didn't know what Darius had in mind, but it felt like the man didn't see the urgency that Drake did about helping Ally and the others trapped in that godforsaken place. To Darius, everything was a calculation, a move on some invisible chessboard where people were pieces to be positioned rather than souls to be saved. The disconnect between them had grown into a chasm that Drake felt in his chest every time he thought about it. Ally was suffering—he knew it in his gut, could feel it like a phantom pain in his own body—and yet the president of the Iron Requiem MC seemed content to wait, to scheme, to let the days slide by while Drake's nerves frayed to the breaking point.

Now he was tired, angry, and frustrated, a dangerous combination that left him snapping at Bunny when she tried to bring him food or ask how he was holding up. He'd apologize later, he always did, but the tension coiled in his shoulders like a live wire. He paced around the small camper where he'd been staying, his heavy boots thudding against the thin carpet, each step echoing the rhythm of his racing thoughts. The RV park was quiet this time of day, most of the residents at work or hiding from the afternoon heat in their air-conditioned units, but Drake barely noticed the stillness outside. His mind was filled with images of Ally's face, of the other girls still trapped in those sterile hallways, of the things that might be happening to them while he stood here doing nothing.

Finally, when the summons came, it arrived in the form of a terse text message from Darius himself: Clubhouse. Now. Drake stared at the screen for a long moment, his thumb hovering over the reply button before he simply shoved the phone into his pocket and grabbed his keys. He'd been waiting for this moment, praying that Darius had finally put together a plan, had finally understood the weight of what Drake had been telling him about Butterfly Academy and the horrors that occurred within its walls.

He wasted no time in getting over there, practically bursting out of the camper door and into the humid afternoon air. The Iron Requiem MC clubhouse wasn't far from the small RV park that Bunny rented a space in for her camper—maybe a fifteen-minute walk if you took the shortcut through the old lumber yard—and in his current state of agitation, Drake didn't even bother to ride his motorcycle. The physical exertion of walking fast, of letting his long legs eat up the distance, helped to channel some of the nervous energy that had been building for days. His boots kicked up dust on the unpaved path, and he could feel his heart hammering against his ribs, not from the mild exertion but from anticipation.

He was sure this was the moment when a plan would finally be revealed to him, a strategy for how they were going to rescue Ally and burn that place to the ground. He'd rehearsed what he would say, how he would volunteer to be on the front line, how he would make Darius understand that he couldn't wait another day. The scenarios played out in his mind like a film reel—breaching the doors, getting the girls out, watching the building crumble behind them as they rode away.

But when he walked into the clubhouse, pushing through the heavy steel door with the Iron Requiem skull-and-wings emblem welded to the front, the atmosphere was all wrong. Instead of the tense, focused energy of men preparing for a mission, Drake was met with the casual languor of a typical afternoon. The air inside was thick with cigarette smoke and the smell of cheap beer, the ceiling fans turning lazily overhead and doing little to disperse the haze. Crew members lounged around the bar, their weathered faces relaxed as they passed bottles back and forth, smoke curling from their lips in lazy spirals. The sound of a cue ball cracking against its fellows rang out from the back corner, where prospects and patched members alike leaned over the green felt of the billiards table, placing bets and talking shit and there, in the center of it all, was Darius.

The president of the Iron Requiem stood near the bar with his second-in-command, Macon, the two of them sharing some private joke that sent Darius's head tipping back in genuine laughter, his gold tooth catching the fluorescent light. He looked comfortable, at ease, the picture of a man without a care in the world. The contrast between Darius's relaxed posture and Drake's own coiled tension made something cold settle in Drake's stomach.

Finally, after what felt like an eternity of Drake standing there in the doorway, Darius noticed him. The president's eyes found his across the room, and that familiar, infuriating smirk spread across his face—the one that said he knew something you didn't, the one that made Drake want to put his fist through the nearest wall.

"Ah, Grudge," Darius called out, his voice carrying easily over the ambient noise of the clubhouse. He used the nickname he'd given Drake since the prospect had first come to the MC looking for sanctuary, a name meant to remind everyone that Drake carried his past like a burden, that he never forgot a slight or a debt. "Glad you could grace us with your presence."

Drake didn't like the nickname. It made him sound like a petulant child holding onto old grievances rather than a man with legitimate grievances against a system that had tried to break him. But he didn't argue about it. Not here, not now, not when he needed Darius's cooperation more than he needed his pride. He rolled his eyes instead, a small defiance, and crossed the room with long strides that ate up the distance between them.

"You called for me, Grim," Drake said, using Darius's own road name, the one he'd earned back in his days running guns through the valley when he'd left a trail of bodies that needed a requiem. "What's up?

Darius's smile widened, becoming something almost predatory, and he exchanged a glance with Macon that made Drake's skin prickle with unease. "Macon, Ruben, and Cole got a special delivery today," Darius said, his voice dropping to a conspiratorial tone that did nothing to ease Drake's growing sense of dread.

Drake scowled, confusion knitting his brow. A special delivery? What the hell did that have to do with Ally? With the rescue mission he thought they were planning? "What kind of delivery?" he asked, but Darius was already moving, already gesturing for Drake to follow.

"Come," Darius said, gesturing toward an open space near the center of the room, away from the tables and the bar. "Stand with me while they bring it in."

Drake reluctantly did as he was told, his boots feeling heavy as he positioned himself beside the club president. Every instinct he had was screaming that something was wrong, that this wasn't the conversation he'd been expecting, but he forced himself to remain still, to wait, to see where this was going. Darius nodded to Macon, and the vice president immediately stepped out through the side door, his heavy boots echoing on the concrete, with Ruben and Cole falling into step behind him.

The minutes that followed were some of the longest of Drake's life. He stood there in the middle of the clubhouse, feeling exposed and foolish, while the other club members continued their conversations around him, oblivious to the tension coiling tighter and tighter in Drake's chest. He could hear the low rumble of a diesel engine outside, the sound of a large van or truck pulling up to the side entrance, and then the scrape of metal on metal as doors were opened.

When they came back in, Drake's world tilted on its axis.

Macon entered first, his massive shoulders filling the doorway, followed by Ruben and Cole flanking three figures that made Drake's blood run cold. They were young women—girls, really—dressed in the distinctive uniforms of Butterfly Academy: the pale blue blouses with the white Peter Pan collars, the gray pleated skirts that fell to just above the knee, the sensible black shoes. But it was the way they moved that told the real story. They shuffled forward with their heads down, their shoulders hunched, their movements synchronized in a way that spoke of training and fear rather than coordination. They were directed to stand directly in front of Darius and Drake, forming a neat little row like dolls on display, and they kept their heads down, their eyes fixed firmly on the scuffed concrete floor, avoiding eye contact with the men surrounding them.

For a moment—a brief, hopeful, stupid moment—Drake wondered if Darius had somehow rescued them without him knowing. Maybe this was the plan, maybe they'd already struck, and these were survivors, freed from that hellhole and brought here for safekeeping.

His heart leaped at the possibility, and he took an involuntary step forward, his hand reaching out—but he soon realized that was wishful thinking. The girls weren't relieved. They weren't celebrating their freedom or looking around with the dazed gratitude of the rescued. They were trembling. He could see it in the way their hands clutched at their skirts, in the way their knees knocked together slightly, in the way they held themselves so still, as if movement might invite punishment.

"Do you like them, Grudge?" Darius asked, his voice rich with amusement and something darker, something that made Drake want to be sick.

"What is this, Grim?" Drake asked, his voice coming out rougher than he intended, edged with a horror he couldn't quite hide.

Darius stepped forward, circling the three girls like a shark circling wounded fish. He reached out and lifted the chin of the one in the middle—a petite brunette with tear tracks staining her cheeks—and she flinched but didn't pull away, her eyes wide and glassy with shock or drugs or both. "Well, you told me all about that school you grew up in," Darius explained, his tone conversational, as if he were discussing the weather or the price of gas. "All about how they train the girls there to be obedient, to be useful, to know their place. And after giving it a lot of thought, I decided that we could use some obedient women around here."

Drake nearly choked, his hand going to his own throat as if he could physically hold back the bile rising there. "I wanted to rescue them, Grim," Drake said, his voice cracking with the effort of keeping it level. "Tear the place down and make the people responsible for its existence pay for their crimes. That's what I told you. That's what I've been telling you for days."

"Please tell me you didn't make a deal with Harold to have these girls brought here..." Drake said, and even as the words left his mouth, he knew the answer. He could see it in the way Darius's eyes lit up, in the satisfaction that radiated off the man like heat.

Darius grinned, and it was the grin of a man who had just won a bet, the grin of a predator who had cornered his prey.

"Of course I did," he said simply, as if it were the most obvious thing in the world. " He assured me that these three will be perfect for us here at Iron Requiem. Top of their class in obedience training, he said. They'll do whatever I tell them to, and they won't argue or refuse." Darius turned back to Drake, and for a moment, something almost like sincerity entered his voice. "I admire what he's doing, Grudge. Creating order in a chaotic world. Taking girls who might have ended up useless and giving them purpose. And you will too, once you see how well they fit in here."

Drake felt the anger boil up inside him, a white-hot rage that started in his gut and spread outward until his vision blurred at the edges. He wanted to scream, to grab Darius by his leather cut and slam him against the wall, to make him understand that this wasn't order, this was slavery, that these weren't willing recruits but broken children. But he didn't want to scare the girls any more than they already were. He could see them out of the corner of his eye, still standing there in their perfect rows, still trembling, and he knew that losing control now would only make their trauma worse.

"Fucking bastard!" Drake exclaimed, the words torn from his throat like a physical wound. He turned on his heel, unable to look at Darius's smug face for another second, unable to look at the girls and see Ally's face superimposed over theirs, and then he stomped out of the MC without looking back. The heavy steel door slammed shut behind him with a sound like a gunshot, but he kept walking, his long strides carrying him away from the clubhouse and the horrors within, his hands shaking with the effort of not putting his fist through the first thing he saw.

The afternoon sun hit him like a physical blow, blinding after the dim interior, but he didn't slow down. He walked without direction, without purpose, his mind a whirlwind of betrayal and fury and the sickening realization that he had been a fool to think Darius would ever be the kind of man who rescued people. The Iron Requiem wasn't a salvation. It was just another cage, and Darius was just another warden wearing a different uniform and Drake had nowhere else to go.

Chapter Twenty-Four

Drake stormed into the camper with the force of a hurricane making landfall, his shoulder hitting the flimsy aluminum door with enough momentum to send it crashing against its frame. The slam was deafening in the small space, a sharp crack of sound that made the entire structure shudder on its cinder block supports. The thin walls rattled in their tracks, causing the small collection of glass figurines on Bunny's windowsill to dance and clink together like wind chimes in a storm. The hanging light fixture above the dinette swayed wildly, casting erratic shadows that spun across the paneled interior.

It startled Bunny, who had been sitting at the narrow fold-down table with a mug of coffee and a battered paperback novel. She jumped visibly, her whole body jerking upright, and the book slipped from her fingers to hit the floor with a soft thud. Coffee sloshed over the rim of her mug, staining the pages and her fingers with dark liquid she didn't bother to wipe away. Her eyes—wide and brown and framed by the brown bangs she'd been growing out—snapped toward the entrance with the alert fear of someone who had learned long ago that loud noises often preceded danger.

"Whoa..." Bunny breathed out, pressing one hand to her chest as if to calm her racing heart. She set the mug down with trembling fingers and rose from her seat, her movements cautious, measured, the way you might approach a wounded animal that could turn vicious without warning. She'd seen Drake angry before—she'd seen him furious, actually, during the months he'd been crashing in her spare bunk—but this was something else entirely. This was rage incarnate, barely contained by skin and will alone. "What's got you in such a rage, Grudge?"

"Don't call me that!" Drake exploded, the words tearing from his throat like shrapnel. He spun toward her, his face flushed crimson beneath his tan, the veins standing out in his neck like cords ready to snap. His hands were clenched at his sides, the knuckles white and bloodless, and she could see the muscles in his jaw working as he ground his teeth together with enough force to make the tendon in his temple jump. "That bastard isn't a friend! He talks about loyalty to the crew and how we stick together no matter what but downright betrayed me!"

He punctuated each word with a gesture, his fists rising and falling in the cramped space between them, and Bunny had to step back to avoid being hit by the wild arc of his arm. Drake began to pace, three steps to the tiny kitchenette, three steps back to the door, his heavy boots making the floor flex and groan beneath his weight. The camper felt even smaller than usual, the air suddenly too thin, too hot, charged with the electricity of his fury.

"I'm sorry, Drake," Bunny said softly, stepping closer to him despite the warning signs, despite the way his body language screamed at her to keep her distance. She reached out, tentative, her fingers hovering in the air between them before she made contact. She touched his chest, flattening her palm against the hard plane of his pecs, feeling the thunderous hammering of his heart beneath the thin cotton of his t-shirt. The heat radiating off his skin was intense, feverish, as if the anger burning inside him had raised his body temperature to dangerous levels. "Grim does whatever he thinks is best for the MC and..."

"But he promised!" Drake cut her off, his voice cracking on the word, and Bunny saw something break behind his eyes—a fissure in the wall of rage that revealed the hurt, the betrayal underneath. He stopped pacing abruptly and turned to face her fully, and she could see that his eyes were glassy, bright with unshed tears that he would never let fall. "And getting girls from the academy after I explained to him what it is and what they do is what he thinks is best?" Drake asked, his voice dropping to something raw and wounded, more devastating than any shout. "After he promised he would help me rescue them?"

He laughed then, a harsh, broken sound that held no humor whatsoever. "I told him everything, Bunny. I told him about the conditioning, about the 'training' they put us through, about the way they break you down until you're nothing but a shell that follows orders. I told him about the basement, about the isolation rooms, about the way they punish you for having thoughts of your own." Drake's hands were shaking now, the anger giving way to something more desperate, more despairing. He dragged his hand over his head, pressing into it until his scalp must have screamed in protest. "And he looked me in the eye and he said he understood. He said we'd get them out. He said we'd burn that place to the ground."

Drake turned away from her, bracing his hands against the small kitchen counter, his head hanging low between his shoulders. His breathing was ragged, audible, each exhale a struggle. "I can't be in Iron Requiem if that's what they're about," he said quietly, the words muffled but clear enough in the silence that followed his outburst. "I can't be part of that. I won't be."

He straightened up, squaring his shoulders, and when he turned back to her, his face was set in the hard lines of resolve. "I'll be out of here before dawn," Drake said. "I'll pack my bag, I'll take my bike, and

I'll be gone. And then I'm going to go to the first police station I find and get help for those girls before I go back and get Ally out of the academy." His voice softened when he said the name, became almost gentle, weighted with a guilt that Bunny knew had been eating him alive since he'd escaped and she hadn't. "I can't keep letting her down. I left her there once. I won't do it again."

Bunny felt her stomach drop at his words, felt the familiar cold grip of fear that had been her constant companion since she'd first run from the MC and then, foolishly, come crawling back when she'd had nowhere else to go. She stepped closer again, her hand finding his chest once more, but this time she used it to push, to make him look at her, to make him understand the gravity of what he was suggesting.

"Drake, you can't just leave," Bunny said, and her voice was urgent now, low and intense. She glanced toward the small window as if afraid of being overheard, even though they were alone in the camper, even though the nearest neighbor was three spaces down and probably too drunk to notice anything. "Darius won't let you."

"The fuck he won't," Drake shot back, but there was less certainty in his voice now, a hesitation that hadn't been there before.

"I don't give a shit," he continued, trying to reclaim that certainty, trying to convince himself as much as her. "He can't stop me. I'll ride until I find a town with a sheriff's department, with state troopers, with anyone who will listen. Those girls in there—" He gestured vaguely toward the clubhouse, though it was miles away now. "—they're victims, Bunny. They're not property. They're not 'obedient women' for his crew to use. They're kids who've been tortured and brainwashed, and I am not going to stand by and watch Darius turn the Iron Requiem into another Butterfly Academy."

"He'll kill you," Bunny said flatly, the words falling between them like stones into still water. She saw Drake freeze, saw the way his throat bobbed as he swallowed hard. "Drake, I'm not exaggerating. I'm not trying to scare you into staying. I'm telling you the truth because I've seen it happen." Her hand was still on his chest, and she could feel his heartbeat stutter, could feel the way his breath caught in his lungs. "Darius doesn't let anyone just leave without his permission. You know the rules. Once you're in, you're in for life, unless he decides otherwise. And if you go to the cops?" She shook her head slowly, her eyes never leaving his. "If you threaten the club, threaten to expose what he's doing? He will make sure you wind up in a ditch somewhere nobody will ever find you. Or worse—he'll make sure you wind up back at the academy, delivered to Harold with a bow on top, and you'll never see daylight again."

Drake looked at her then, really looked at her, and saw the truth written in the lines around her eyes, in the way she held herself so carefully, as if she were still waiting for a blow to fall. He knew she was serious. He knew that tone in her voice, that particular flatness that came from having seen things you couldn't unsee, from having survived things that should have broken you. She knew from personal experience—he understood that implicitly, though he didn't press her for information. Whatever had happened to her in her time with the MC, whatever had made her come back after she'd tried to leave once before, it was written in the language of her body, in the way she flinched at sudden movements and checked locks three times before sleeping.

"So what?" Drake asked, but the fight had gone out of his voice, replaced by a weary desperation that was somehow more heartbreaking than his rage had been. He sank down onto the small bench seat that ran along the side of the camper, his elbows on his knees, his head in his hands. "I'm just supposed to stay and go along with whatever he does after he betrayed me? I'm supposed to smile and nod while those girls are... while they're..." He couldn't finish the sentence, couldn't make himself say the words.

Bunny moved to sit beside him, the vinyl cushion compressing under their combined weight. The camper was dimming around them as the sun began to set, painting the interior in shades of orange and purple that filtered through the thin curtains. She didn't touch him now, didn't try to offer physical comfort that he wouldn't accept. Instead, she sat close enough that he could feel her presence, solid and real, an anchor in the storm.

"It's a test," Bunny said quietly, her voice barely above a whisper. She was staring straight ahead, at the small sink with its mismatched dishes, at the life they'd cobbled together in this tiny space. "He pushes everyone's buttons to see if they will remain loyal or not. It's how he weeds out the weak ones, the ones who can't be trusted. He finds your weakness—your soft spot—and he pokes at it until you bleed, until you either break or prove you're strong enough to take it."

She turned to look at him then, and her eyes were bright in the gathering darkness, fierce with a knowledge that came from hard-won survival. "And trust me, Drake," she said, her voice steady now, certain. "You don't want to fail if you ever hope to get out of here alive. Because the only way out of Iron Requiem—the only way that's not in a body bag—is through Darius's good graces. You have to play the game. You have to eat the shit he feeds you and smile while you do it, until he trusts you enough to let you walk away."

Drake sighed, a long, shuddering exhale that seemed to deflate him, to let out the last of the fight he'd been holding onto. He hated it. He hated every word she'd said, hated the truth of it, hated the system that Darius had built that made prisoners of them all. But he knew she was right. He'd seen it happen to others—prospects who'd tried to leave, members who'd questioned too loudly, people who'd simply disappeared one day and were never spoken of again.

The camper grew darker around them as the sun dipped below the horizon, and Drake sat in the gathering gloom, feeling the weight of his choices pressing down on his chest like a physical burden. He thought of Ally, somewhere in the sterile halls of the academy, waiting for a rescue that wasn't coming. He thought of the three girls Darius had "acquired," their downcast eyes and trembling hands. He thought of his bike outside, of the open road, of freedom that was just an illusion and he hated himself for knowing that, come morning, he would do exactly what Bunny suggested. He would swallow his pride.

He would play the game. He would become the loyal soldier Darius wanted him to be, and he would wait—God help him, he would wait—for a chance that might never come.

"Okay," Drake said finally, the word tasting like ash in his mouth. "Okay. I'll stay."

But even as he said it, he made a silent promise to himself. He would play the game, yes. But he would play it to win. And someday—someday soon—Darius would learn what happened when you pushed a man with a grudge too far.

After standing there for several moments breathing hard, the silence of the camper settling around them like a heavy blanket, Drake began to cool down. The white-hot rage that had been consuming him since he'd walked out of the Iron Requiem clubhouse slowly receded, leaving behind a hollow emptiness that felt almost worse than the anger had been. His shoulders, which had been bunched up near his ears with tension, began to relax, dropping incrementally as his breathing steadied into something approaching normal. He didn't move, though. He remained rooted to the spot just inside the door, his boots planted wide on the thin carpet, his hands hanging loose at his sides but still faintly trembling from the adrenaline that hadn't quite worked its way out of his system.

The light had faded almost completely now, the last orange vestiges of sunset giving way to the deep purple-blue of early evening. The single bulb above the dinette cast a warm, amber glow that didn't quite reach the corners of the small space, leaving pools of shadow that shifted and breathed with the movement of the air. Outside, the RV park was settling into its nighttime routine—the distant sound of a television through thin walls, the occasional bark of a dog, the low rumble of a diesel generator kicking on somewhere down the row.

"You know..." Bunny said, her voice cutting through the quiet in a way that made him turn his head. She was still sitting on the bench seat where she'd joined him, but she'd shifted, turning her body to face him fully. When he locked eyes with her, he saw something there that hadn't been present before—not fear, not caution, but a kind of determined understanding that made his breath catch in his throat. Her brown eyes were darker in the dim light, the pupils blown wide, and there was a softness to her expression that hadn't been there when she'd been warning him about Darius's wrath.

"You've been on edge since you arrived," Bunny continued, her voice dropping to a register that vibrated somewhere low in his gut. It wasn't quite a whisper, but it was intimate nonetheless, meant only for him, for this space they shared. She rose from the bench with a fluid grace that belied the cramped quarters, closing the distance between them in two slow steps. "Tense. Coiled tight. Walking around like you're waiting for someone to hit you."

She reached out, her hand finding his chest again, but this time her touch was different. This wasn't the placating gesture from before, the attempt to calm a wild animal. This was something else entirely—deliberate, purposeful, charged with an electricity that had nothing to do with comfort and everything to do with need. Slowly, deliberately, she moved her hand down his chest, her palm dragging across the fabric of his t-shirt, feeling the hard planes of muscle beneath, the steady thunder of his heart. She traced the ridges of his abs through the thin cotton, each fingertip leaving a trail of heat that seemed to burn through the material and into his skin and stopped at his belt buckle.

She smiled then, a mischievous quirk of her lips that transformed her face from serious to something playful, something hungry. It was a smile that said she knew exactly what she was doing, that she'd been thinking about this for longer than she cared to admit, that she wanted to be the one to break through the walls he'd built so high around himself.

"I'm sure you could use some relief," Bunny said, the words rolling off her tongue with a suggestive weight that made his pulse jump. Without waiting for a response, without giving him a chance to process what was happening, she casually began to unfasten his belt. Her fingers were nimble, practiced, working the leather through the metal buckle with a soft clink that sounded impossibly loud in the quiet space. He didn't stop her. He stood there, frozen, watching as she tugged the belt loose in one smooth motion and tossed it onto the ground, where it landed with a muffled thud against the thin carpet.

"Bunny..." Drake said, his voice rough, barely recognizable as his own. It was meant to be a warning, a question, something, but it came out as a rasp that sounded more like encouragement than objection. She looked up at him, her hand already moving to his zipper, her fingers finding the metal tab and drawing it down with agonizing slowness. The sound of the teeth separating was a hiss in the darkness. "You don't have to..." Drake managed, though his body was betraying him, responding to her proximity, to the warmth of her breath through his clothes, to the promise in her eyes but she shook her head, that smirk still playing at the corners of her mouth, and there was something fierce in her expression now, something that brooked no argument.

"I want to," Bunny said simply, and there was no mistaking the truth in her voice. This wasn't obligation. This wasn't pity. This was desire, plain and simple, the kind that had been building between them for weeks of close quarters and shared silences, of him sleeping in her spare bunk and her pretending not to notice the way he looked at her when he thought she wasn't paying attention.

She hooked her fingers into the waistband of his jeans and tugged, the denim sliding down over his hips with a soft whisper of fabric against skin. He hadn't been wearing underwear—the laundry situation in the camper had been dire for days—and his erection sprang free as soon as the constraint was gone, jutting proud and heavy against his stomach in the dim light. The cool air of the camper hit heated flesh, but he barely registered it, too focused on the way Bunny's eyes went dark with appreciation, the way her lips parted in a silent gasp.

"Impressive," Bunny murmured, and there was genuine admiration in her tone, a hunger that made him feel powerful despite the vulnerability of his position, pants around his thighs, heart laid bare. She didn't waste time with teasing, with building anticipation. She simply leaned forward, her choppy brown hair falling forward to frame her face and took him into her mouth.

The heat and wet suction of it hit him like a physical blow, his knees buckling slightly as a groan tore itself from his throat, raw and unguarded. He hadn't expected this—hadn't let himself hope for it, hadn't thought he deserved it after the mess he'd made of everything, after the way he'd snapped at her earlier in his rage. But Bunny seemed determined to wash all of that away, to replace his anger with sensation, his frustration with pleasure. She worked him with lips and tongue and the occasional scrape of teeth, her head moving in a steady rhythm that had his hands flying to her shoulders, gripping hard enough to bruise, needing something to anchor himself to reality.

It felt good—God, it felt good—and even though he was still furious at Darius for betraying him, furious at himself for being trapped in this impossible situation, furious at the world for being so goddamn unfair, he would allow himself this. He would allow himself to enjoy it for tonight, to be selfish, to take what she was offering without guilt or reservation. Tomorrow would bring its own battles, its own impossible choices. But tonight, in this cramped camper with the woman who had seen him at his worst and hadn't run, he would simply feel.

He watched Bunny's head moving back and forth over his shaft, the sight almost as overwhelming as the sensation itself—the way her lips stretched around him, the way her throat worked, the way her hand came up to grip what she couldn't take and then she backed off him with a wet sound that should have been obscene but was instead the most erotic thing he'd ever heard, and she looked up at him with those dark eyes, her mouth swollen and glistening, and she moved lower.

She suckled his balls one by one, taking each into the warmth of her mouth, letting her tongue glide over the prickly red stubble with a delicacy that contrasted sharply with the roughness of his need, and the sensation was so intense, so overwhelming, that he felt himself start to grow weak in the knees. His legs trembled, his grip on her shoulders tightening, and he knew that if he didn't move, didn't take control, he was going to collapse right there in the middle of her kitchenette.

"Bed," he managed to grit out, his voice sounding like gravel scraping over glass. "Now."

She understood immediately, reading his body language, the desperation in his tone. She guided him, her hand wrapping around his wrist and pulling him the few steps to the sleeping area, the narrow bunk that took up the back third of the camper. She'd made it that morning, he noticed distantly, the quilt pulled tight, the pillows fluffed, and he felt a surge of gratitude for her domesticity, for the normalcy of it, for the way she made this place feel like a home even when his life was falling apart.

He laid down on his back, the mattress dipping under his weight, and she followed him, crawling up between his legs with a predatory grace that made his breath hitch in his chest. She happily continued where she'd left off, her mouth finding him again, working him with renewed enthusiasm now that she had better leverage, now that she could use her hands as well. She varied her rhythm, alternating between long, slow pulls and quick, teasing flicks of her tongue, and he could feel the pressure building at the base of his spine, the familiar tightening that meant he was close.

But he didn't want to finish like this. He didn't want to be passive, to be the one receiving. He needed to be active, to take, to claim some small piece of control in a world that had stripped him of every other kind. Just as he was teetering on the edge, his hips bucking involuntarily, his hands fisted in her hair, he guided her to her feet with gentle but firm pressure.

She stood there for a moment, looking down at him, her chest heaving, her lips parted, and then she began to undress herself with an efficiency that spoke of practice. She pulled her tank top over her head, revealing a simple cotton bra that she dispatched just as quickly, her breasts spilling free, pale and perfect in the dim light. She shimmied out of her shorts and underwear in one motion, kicking them aside, and then she was bare before him, all soft curves and sharp angles, the scars of her past visible but not defining, a map of survival written on her skin.

She swung a leg over his hips, positioning herself above him, her heat hovering just out of reach, her hand reaching down to guide him. But before she could take him inside her, before she could sink down and envelop him in that wet heat, he moved. With a surge of strength that surprised even himself, he flipped her onto her back, pinning her beneath him on the narrow mattress, and entered her with a hard thrust that drove the air from both their lungs.

She moaned loudly, the sound echoing off the thin walls of the camper, unrestrained and primal, and he didn't pause, didn't give her time to adjust. He set a punishing pace, thrusting deeply, angling his hips to hit the spot that made her cry out, her nails digging crescents into his shoulders. He wasn't interested in taking things slow tonight—couldn't, even if he'd wanted to. There was too much pent-up energy, too much frustration and fear and fury that needed an outlet, and Bunny was offering herself as the vessel for all of it.

She could handle it. He knew that from the way she urged him on, her legs wrapping around his waist to pull him deeper, her hips meeting his thrust for thrust, her voice breaking on his name and begging for more. "Harder," she gasped, her head thrown back against the pillow, her throat exposed and vulnerable. "Don't hold back, Drake. Give me everything."

So he did. He lost himself in the rhythm, in the slap of skin against skin, in the way the camper rocked slightly on its foundations with the force of their movements. The sounds of their pleasure filled the small space—her moans, his grunts, the wet slide of their joining, the creak of the bedframe protesting beneath them. It was raw and real and exactly what he needed, a reminder that he was alive, that he could feel good things even in the midst of the darkness, that there was still something worth fighting for.

Several minutes passed—could have been hours, could have been seconds, time lost all meaning in the haze of sensation—and he felt her begin to tighten around him, her internal muscles fluttering, her breath coming in short, sharp gasps that signaled she was close. He shifted his angle slightly, grinding against her with each thrust, and that was all it took. Her orgasm overtook her with a violence that made her scream his name, the sound tearing from her throat, her back arching off the bed, her body shuddering beneath him as wave after wave of pleasure crashed through her.

He pulled out as she continued to pulse around nothing, her hands scrabbling at his back, her eyes glazed and unfocused. He took himself in hand, stroking twice, three times, and then he was coming too, spilling himself across the bedsheets in long, hot pulses that seemed to drain the last of the tension from his body. He let out a long, shuddering sigh, his forehead dropping to rest against her shoulder, his breathing ragged and loud in the sudden quiet.

For a long moment, they lay there like that, tangled together, the sweat cooling on their skin, the camper dark and still around them. He didn't know how much he'd needed that—not just the physical release, but the connection, the intimacy, the reminder that he wasn't alone in this. Bunny's hand came up to stroke through his smooth head, her fingers gentle now, soothing, and he felt something loosen in his chest that had been knotted tight for days.

Tomorrow would bring its own horrors. Tomorrow he would have to face Darius again, would have to decide whether to play the game or make a run for it, would have to live with the knowledge that Ally was still trapped and he was doing nothing to save her. But for now, in this moment, with Bunny's warmth surrounding him and the scent of her filling his lungs, he allowed himself to simply be. To rest. To gather his strength for the battles yet to come.

Chapter Twenty-Five

Drake was awake long before the first hint of dawn crept over the horizon.

Sleep had come only in short, restless stretches, each one interrupted by memories of the Butterfly Academy, Ally's frightened face, and Darius' calm expression as he dismissed everything Drake had fought for. By the time he finally gave up trying to sleep, the digital clock beside the camper bed read a little after four in the morning.

The tiny camper was quiet.

Outside, the RV park was still wrapped in darkness. The occasional chirp of a cricket and the distant hum of traffic were the only sounds drifting through the thin walls.

Drake quietly zipped his worn backpack shut. He paused for a moment and looked around the cramped living space that Bunny had generously shared with him over the past several months.

His gaze shifted toward the small bed in the back of the camper. Bunny lay fast asleep, curled onto her side beneath a blanket that had become hopelessly tangled around her naked form sometime during the night. A few strands of her short brown hair had fallen across her face, and her breathing was slow and steady.

She looked peaceful.

Drake felt a pang of guilt. He knew exactly what she would say if she woke up and saw him standing there with his backpack slung over his shoulder. She would try to talk him out of leaving. She would tell him to think it through.

She would remind him how dangerous it could be and part of him knew she'd only be trying to protect him but his mind was made up.

He couldn't stay.

Not after what had happened at the clubhouse. Not after watching Darius turn his back on everything Drake believed was right. Iron Requiem wasn't the family he'd hoped it would become. It was time to walk away.

He wasn't planning to disappear without a word, though. Darius deserved to hear it from him directly. Drake intended to look him in the eye and tell him exactly why he was leaving whether Darius liked it or not.

He quietly slipped his arms through the straps of his backpack and adjusted its weight. Before turning away, he looked at Bunny one last time.

"Thanks," he whispered so softly he barely heard himself. "Take care of yourself."

She didn't stir. Satisfied that she was still asleep, Drake carefully crossed the camper. He eased the lock open, grasped the handle, and slowly pulled the door toward him. The hinges gave a faint squeak. He froze. Bunny shifted slightly beneath the blankets, letting out a sleepy sigh before settling again.

Drake waited another few seconds. When she remained asleep, he quietly stepped outside and eased the door shut behind him until the latch clicked with barely a sound.

Cool morning air greeted him. He drew in a deep breath, letting it fill his lungs before slowly exhaling. The sky overhead was still dark, though a faint gray band had begun forming along the eastern horizon.

The RV park was silent.

Most of the campers were dark, their occupants still asleep. A light breeze rustled the leaves of a nearby tree. Drake adjusted the straps on his backpack and started walking.

He deliberately left his motorcycle where it was. He wasn't running. Not yet. There was no need to roar out of the park and wake everyone before sunrise. Besides, he needed time to think.

His boots crunched softly across the gravel as he made his way toward the road. A few blocks away, the familiar glow of a twenty-four-hour diner sign cut through the darkness. Its neon lights reflected off the windows, promising hot coffee and breakfast to the handful of early risers passing through town.

Drake headed straight for it.

The bell above the diner's door jingled softly as he stepped inside. Warm air wrapped around him immediately, carrying the comforting aromas of fresh coffee, bacon, pancakes, and sizzling hash browns.

Compared to the cool darkness outside, it felt almost welcoming. Only a few customers occupied the booths. An elderly couple quietly shared breakfast near the window. A truck driver sat alone at the counter reading the newspaper while absently stirring cream into his coffee.

Soft country music drifted from an old radio somewhere behind the kitchen pass-through. A tired-looking waitress looked up and offered him a friendly smile.

"Morning."

"Mornin'," Drake replied quietly.

"Just one?"

He nodded. She grabbed a menu and handed it to him, though he barely looked at it as she led him to a booth near the back.

"What can I get you to drink?"

"Coffee. Black."

"You got it."

A minute later she returned with a steaming mug. Drake wrapped both hands around it, welcoming the warmth. He stared into the dark liquid without taking a sip.

His thoughts immediately drifted back to Darius. He replayed the conversation in the clubhouse over and over. Every word. Every expression. Every moment. The betrayal still burned.

He wasn't sure exactly how he was going to say it when he saw Darius. Part of him wanted to yell. Another part wanted to simply hand over his prospect cut, turn around, and walk away forever. Neither option felt satisfying. He wanted Darius to understand why.

He wanted him to know that Drake couldn't stand beside someone whose choices conflicted so deeply with his own sense of right and wrong.

The waitress returned with her notepad.

"You ready to order, honey?"

Drake blinked, realizing he'd forgotten to open the menu.

"Uh...yeah, I'll take the bacon, eggs, hash browns, and toast."

"Coming right up."

She disappeared toward the kitchen. Drake finally lifted the mug and took a long drink of coffee. It was hot and bitter. Exactly what he needed.

He looked out the window. Beyond the glass, the eastern sky was beginning to glow with the first colors of sunrise. A new day was beginning. Whatever happened after breakfast...there would be no turning back.

The rumble of Drake's motorcycle echoed across the Iron Requiem clubhouse parking lot before fading into silence.

He killed the engine and sat for a moment, gripping the handlebars. The morning air was cool, but it did nothing to calm the anger simmering beneath his skin.

Breakfast had helped him think but it hadn't changed his mind.

He climbed off the Harley, slung his backpack over one shoulder, and walked toward the clubhouse entrance with steady, deliberate steps. The familiar smell of cigarette smoke and stale beer greeted him as he stepped inside. Conversation continued for another second before several heads turned.

A few members nodded. Others simply watched. Darius stood near the bar, coffee mug in one hand, laughing with Macon, Ruben, and Cole. When he noticed Drake, his smile widened.

"Morning, Grudge."

Drake didn't return the smile.

"We need to talk."

Something in his voice caused the room to grow noticeably quieter. Darius set his mug on the bar.

"Sounds serious."

"It is."

The two men stood facing one another in the center of the clubhouse. No one else spoke. Drake took a slow breath.

"I'm done."

Darius raised an eyebrow.

"Done?"

"I came here because I thought Iron Requiem stood for something, I believed you and I believed your word, you said this club was family, you said loyalty mattered."

"It does."

Drake shook his head.

"Not the kind of loyalty I'm willing to live by."

He met Darius' gaze without flinching. "I don't agree with the way you run this club; I don't agree with the decisions you've made and I don't want any part of it anymore."

The silence became almost oppressive. Darius regarded him for several long moments. Finally he spoke.

"You don't simply walk away from Iron Requiem."

Drake's expression never changed.

"I'm walking away."

"No." Darius' voice hardened. "Nobody leaves unless I say they can."

"I'm not asking."

Drake slipped the prospect cut from his shoulders and laid it carefully on a nearby table.

"It belongs to Iron Requiem; it never belonged to me." He took a step backward. "I'm leaving."

Darius' eyes shifted briefly toward Macon. The movement was almost imperceptible. Macon understood immediately and he stepped into Drake's path.

"So that's it?" Macon asked. "You think you can insult Grim and stroll out?"

Drake sighed.

"I don't want to fight anybody."

Cole moved to one side. Ruben to the other. The three men now stood between Drake and the clubhouse door.

"You've got one chance," Macon said quietly. "Stay."

"No." Drake answered without hesitation.

Macon reached for his shoulder and Drake instinctively knocked the hand away. The movement sparked the confrontation.

Macon lunged first. Drake sidestepped, and the two collided shoulder to shoulder. Before Drake could regain his balance, Ruben caught him around the waist. Cole grabbed for his arm.

The four men stumbled into a nearby table, sending cards and beer bottles crashing onto the floor. Chairs scraped loudly as club members hurried out of the way.

Darius remained exactly where he was. Watching. Not cheering or intervening. Simply observing. Drake planted his boots against the floor and twisted hard, breaking Ruben's grip long enough to shove him backward.

Macon charged again. A heavy collision sent both men sprawling against the edge of a pool table. Pain shot through Drake's shoulder, but adrenaline drowned it out. Cole grabbed his backpack strap and the old fabric tore free with a loud rip. Drake spun away before anyone could regain a solid hold on him. For a brief second, an opening appeared. He didn't waste it.

Drake backed away from the group, breathing hard. His eyes never left Darius.

"I meant what I said." His voice was steady despite the pounding of his heart. "I won't be part of this."

Without another word, he turned and strode toward the exit. No one followed immediately. The clubhouse remained silent behind him.

Outside, he crossed the parking lot without looking back. He swung onto his motorcycle, started the engine, and paused only long enough to glance once toward the clubhouse doors. Whatever future he'd imagined with Iron Requiem was over. He eased the bike into gear and rolled out of the lot and as the clubhouse disappeared behind him, Drake felt no triumph.

Only uncertainty. He was alone again but he knew that he had to get as far away from there as possible because there was no doubt in his mind that they would be coming after him.

Chapter Twenty-Six

The first few days after he escaped Iron Requiem, Drake convinced himself that he had simply gotten lucky.

He rode until the fuel gauge dipped dangerously close to empty, found a nameless roadside motel, paid cash for a room, slept for a handful of restless hours, and left before sunrise. He never stayed anywhere long enough for anyone to notice him. It was the same routine he had followed for years before joining the club, and he hoped it would be enough to disappear once again.

It wasn't.

The first time they found him was only three days later. He had just stepped out of another convenience store carrying a paper cup of burnt coffee and a stale breakfast sandwich when three motorcycles rolled into the parking lot.

He recognized the black and silver cuts immediately.

Iron Requiem.

His stomach dropped. The riders hadn't even removed their helmets before one of them pointed directly at him.

"There he is!"

Drake cursed under his breath.

"So much for breakfast."

He threw the coffee into the nearest trash can, dropped the sandwich onto the seat of his motorcycle, and swung his leg over the Harley in one practiced motion.

The engine roared to life. The other bikers did the same and tires squealed. Drake shot out of the parking lot just as one of the Iron Requiem riders reached for him.

For nearly twenty miles they chased him along twisting back roads before finally giving up. When they disappeared from his mirrors, Drake slowed just enough to breathe again.

"They're serious..." he muttered. He had embarrassed Darius and men like Darius Crowe did not forgive humiliation.

They collected debts. They punished betrayal.

Weeks became months. Months slowly blurred into years. Every town became another temporary stop. Every motel room was nothing more than borrowed shelter.

Drake stopped unpacking his backpack altogether. There wasn't any point. He would be gone before long. He slept with his boots beside the bed. His motorcycle keys stayed in his pocket even while he showered.

Every unfamiliar engine outside made him freeze. Every knock on a motel door made his pulse race. More than once he climbed out bathroom windows just to avoid answering it. Sometimes the men hunting him belonged to Iron Requiem. Sometimes they wore no colors at all.

That was almost worse. Darius had friends, associates, satellite crews, and prospects looking to earn favor and Drake never knew who might recognize his face.

One rainy evening he had barely finished paying for a room when two heavily tattooed bikers walked into the motel office.

He caught sight of one patch. There was no mistake that they were from Iron Requiem. Without saying a word, Drake turned around, walked straight back outside, climbed onto his Harley, and left before the clerk even realized he hadn't collected his room key.

Another time he had almost managed an entire peaceful week working under a fake name repairing farm equipment. The owner had liked him. The old mechanic had even invited him over for Sunday dinner with his family.

Drake almost accepted when a black pickup truck rolled slowly past the garage. Inside sat Macon. The large biker looked directly at Drake through the windshield.

Neither man moved. Neither spoke. Macon simply smiled a cold, patient smile. The kind that promised,

I know where you are.

That night Drake packed without collecting his final paycheck. He left before midnight. The old mechanic never knew why. Drake hated that. He hated leaving decent people wondering what they'd done wrong. He hated never saying goodbye. He hated never allowing anyone close enough to become part of his life but the alternative was worse.

Iron Requiem didn't just punish the people who crossed them. They punished anyone standing beside them and Drake refused to let innocent people pay for his choices.

As the years slipped past, the constant vigilance wore him down. His already restless sleep became even worse. Some nights he managed only two hours before another nightmare dragged him awake. Sometimes they all merged together into one endless nightmare where every road led back to another prison. He would wake soaked in sweat, breathing hard, instinctively reaching for a weapon that wasn't there. Then came the familiar silence.

Another anonymous motel room. Another unfamiliar ceiling. Another day. His red beard grew thicker. New scars joined the old ones. Fine lines appeared around his tired green eyes.

His motorcycle accumulated thousands upon thousands of miles. The Harley remained the only constant companion he had left. He kept it running with spare parts scavenged from junkyards and whatever repairs he could perform himself.

Sometimes he talked to it while tightening bolts or changing the oil. It was ridiculous, he knew that, but machines never lied.

They never betrayed him. They simply carried him forward.

Every once in a while, usually late at night while riding empty highways beneath endless stars, his thoughts drifted back to the people he'd left behind.

Bunny.

He hoped she'd found a better life somehow. Though deep down he doubted Darius would ever allow that.

Donovan. Ambrosia.

He still couldn't understand Donovan's choices. He had replayed those conversations hundreds of times. Looking for something he'd missed. Some explanation but he never found one.

Then there was Ally.

She remained the hardest memory of all. Every year she grew older in his imagination. He tried to picture her. Nine. Ten. Eleven. Twelve. Each birthday he wasn't there to see felt like another personal failure.

He wondered if she still remembered the man who used to make her laugh on long road trips. He wondered if Butterfly Academy had already stripped those memories away. That thought hurt more than any bruise Iron Requiem had ever given him. He had once dreamed of rescuing every child trapped inside those academies.

Now he struggled just to survive long enough to keep the dream alive. Some nights that realization nearly broke him.

Still, every morning he climbed back onto the Harley. Every morning he turned the key. Every morning he rode because as long as he was still breathing...as long as Iron Requiem hadn't caught him...as long as Helena and Harold hadn't won...there was still the smallest chance that one day he would find the people he needed.

One day he would stop running. One day he would ride toward the academies instead of away from those hunting him and when that day finally came, he intended to make sure neither the academies nor Iron Requiem would ever threaten another child again.

Chapter Twenty-Seven

Five years, four months, two weeks, and ten days.

That was how long Iron Requiem had hunted him. Drake knew the exact amount of time because somewhere along the endless miles he had finally started counting.

At first it had been to keep himself sane. Later it became a reminder that he had survived another day. Now it only served as proof of how long he had spent running from a life he never should have joined.

How long he had slept in cheap motels with one eye open. How long he had avoided making friends because anyone close to him became a target. How long he had lived with the constant expectation that every unfamiliar motorcycle engine meant another fight.

It had worn him down. His shoulders ached with exhaustion that sleep could never cure. The lines around his tired green eyes had deepened. The optimism that had once driven him to save Ally and destroy the academies had slowly eroded until all that remained was quiet disappointment.

He had failed.

No matter how many times he tried to tell himself otherwise, that truth never changed. Ally would not be the cheerful little girl learning to read beside Ambrosia anymore.

She had spent than five years inside Butterfly Academy. Five years of Helena's influence. Five years of Harold's twisted teachings. Five years of becoming someone Drake no longer knew. If she was even alive.

That thought hurt more than anything Iron Requiem had ever done to him.

His Harley rumbled beneath him as he coasted to the shoulder of a lonely highway. The engine idled with its familiar vibration while he stared toward the city ahead. Something about it tugged at his memory.

He had been there once. Long ago. He couldn't remember its name. Only the skyline. Tall brick buildings, old warehouses, and church steeples rising above rooftops blackened with age. Everything about it looked worn by decades of weather yet somehow still standing.

Kind of like him.

Drake shut off the motorcycle. Silence settled around him. For a long moment he simply sat there. The breeze drifted across the highway carrying the scent of hot pavement and distant rain.

His hand slipped into his jacket pocket. His fingers wrapped around a crushed cigarette pack. He opened it. One cigarette remained. He stared at it for several seconds before placing it between his lips.

The lighter clicked, the end glowed orange, and he inhaled deeply. Smoke filled his lungs and he held it there. Then slowly released it into the afternoon air.

"I've really gotta quit these..." he muttered to himself.

The thought barely had time to fade before another sound reached him.

Motorcycles. Several of them. His eyes closed. A long, tired sigh escaped him. The engines grew louder. Closer. He didn't even bother looking. He already knew.

A dozen motorcycles rolled onto the shoulder behind him before spreading into a loose semicircle.

Black leather. Silver patches.

Darius pulled up alongside him. His steel-blue eyes met Drake's as he shut off his motorcycle. For several seconds neither man spoke. Drake took another drag from the cigarette.

"You don't quit, do you?" he finally asked, smoke escaping with every word.

Darius smirked.

"I told you years ago," he said calmly. "You don't leave Iron Requiem unless I say so."

Drake laughed quietly. There wasn't any humor in it.

"Yet you've had my people chasing your ass all over the damn country for the last five years." Darius folded his arms. "Which I must say..." His grin widened. "Is an impressive feat, You kept giving them the slip when they'd catch your trail and you'd disappear, but we'd find you again and again, you made us work for it."

Drake shrugged.

"I didn't make you do anything, Grim, you could've forgotten I ever existed, you could've let me walk away."

Darius chuckled.

"Nah, that's not how I do things." He gave a single nod.

It happened instantly. Macon reached Drake first. Ruben grabbed one arm and Cole seized the other. Several more bikers crowded in until Drake disappeared inside a wall of leather and denim.

Strong hands yanked him off the Harley. His boots scraped uselessly across the gravel. Someone drove a shoulder into his ribs. Another twisted his arms behind his back. Within seconds they forced him onto both knees. Gravel bit into his jeans. His cigarette slipped from his lips. It landed beside him, still burning.

He watched the tiny ribbon of smoke curl into the air. Then a boot crushed it flat. Drake coughed once and looked up. That was when he noticed what Darius carried. A thick wooden club.

Homemade. Heavy. Long rusted nails protruded from one end. Several were bent. Dark brown stains surrounded the heads where they had been driven through the wood. Drake knew immediately it had been used before.

His stomach tightened.

"So..." He swallowed. "This is it?"

Darius tilted his head.

"This is what?"

"You're just going to kill me out here in the middle of nowhere?"

A few of the surrounding bikers exchanged uneasy looks. Darius merely shrugged.

"If you die."

Drake frowned.

"If?"

"I've watched you survive a hell of a lot." Darius slowly turned the club in his hands. "You seem pretty resilient and I'd like to see exactly how much you can take."

Uneasy whispers spread through the gathered crew. Someone muttered that this had gone far enough. Another quietly laughed. Darius didn't even glance toward them.

"Enough."

The whispers stopped immediately. Silence returned. Drake lowered his gaze. He didn't fight. He didn't struggle. Didn't even try to stand. There wasn't any point.

"I'm not going to fight you, Grim." His voice sounded strangely calm. "So..." He looked back up. "Just do whatever you're going to do."

Darius's smile widened.

"There he is." He lifted the club. Drake closed his eyes. His breathing slowed.

He thought of Ally. Of Catarina finally going home. Of his father working beneath the hood of a car beside another son. Of mornings eating breakfast with the Stray Sons before everything fell apart. Of Bunny trying to warn him and of all the years he had spent running.

He was tired. So incredibly tired. The wind shifted. Then—more motorcycles. Fast. Very fast. Several engines. They were approaching rapidly. Voices erupted somewhere down the highway.

Someone shouted.

"What the hell—"

Darius didn't hesitate. The club came down. Crack. Agony exploded across Drake's skull. His vision instantly blurred. Stars burst across his eyes and he swayed but somehow remained upright on his knees. Blood ran warm down the side of his face.

A sharp ringing filled both ears. Another impact. Crack. The world tilted violently. The ringing became deafening. Voices surrounded him from every direction. Men shouting. Motorcycles skidding. Someone screaming orders. Someone yelling in anger.

The sounds blended together into meaningless noise. Drake couldn't tell who belonged to Iron Requiem anymore. Everything echoed as though underwater.

He tried to focus. Couldn't. Shapes moved. Boots. Dust. Chrome. Flashes of black leather. Another voice shouted something close by.

Then—the final swing. The nailed club crashed against the side of his head with sickening force. For the briefest instant there was no pain at all. Only darkness rushing toward him.

The voices disappeared, the ringing stopped, and everything went black.

Chapter Twenty-Eight

Drake surfaced slowly from the darkness.

At first there was only pain. It was everywhere.

His head throbbed with a deep, crushing ache that pulsed in time with his heartbeat. Every breath made his ribs complain. His shoulders felt bruised, his neck was stiff, and even his jaw hurt when he tried to move it.

It felt as though a semi truck had run him over, backed up, and then thrown him off the side of a mountain for good measure.

A low groan escaped him before he even realized he was awake. Something warm and damp rested gently against his forehead. The cloth moved in slow, careful circles, wiping away sweat that had gathered there.

"Man," a familiar voice said with a quiet chuckle, "you sure have a hard head."

Drake frowned. He knew that voice. Somewhere. He just couldn't place it. His eyelids felt impossibly heavy as he forced them open. Everything was blurry.

The ceiling above him swam in and out of focus. Shadows shifted around the room. His stomach rolled unpleasantly.

"Easy," the voice continued. "Jethro is certain you have a skull fracture, but he says it doesn't appear you've got any internal bleeding."

Drake blinked several times.

"Jethro?" he croaked. His throat burned and his tongue felt swollen. His mouth was so dry it seemed to be full of cotton. "Who's... Jethro?"

"Get him some water."

Footsteps hurried away. A moment later he heard a faucet running somewhere nearby. Water splashed into a glass. More footsteps approached and gentle hands slid behind his shoulders.

"Easy now," someone said softly. They carefully helped him sit just high enough without jarring his injuries. A cool glass touched his lips. "Small sips."

Drake obeyed. The cold water felt like heaven. He drank slowly, swallowing one careful mouthful after another until the burning in his throat eased.

He let out a long sigh.

"Thanks..."

The hands lowered him carefully back onto the mattress. He closed his eyes for another few seconds before opening them again. This time his vision steadied.

The room slowly came into focus. It wasn't a hospital. Several old double beds lined both sides of the room. Some were occupied by sleeping men. Others sat empty with rumpled blankets tossed across them. At the far end stood a small bathroom with its door hanging halfway open.

The air carried the unmistakable smells of cigarette smoke, stale beer, leather, motor oil, and antiseptic. It was oddly comforting. Certainly more welcoming than the sterile scent of a hospital.

"Where am I?" Drake asked quietly. His eyes drifted toward the man sitting beside the bed.

Dark hair, familiar tattoos, blue eyes and a crooked grin. Recognition struck almost instantly.

"Viper?..."

The man smirked.

"Heh, yeah."

Drake stared at him for several seconds. His brain struggled to catch up. It had been years.

"Welcome to Venom Bite." There was unmistakable pride in Viper's voice. "My MC." He leaned back comfortably in the chair. "I own it."

Drake let out a weak laugh before immediately regretting it as pain shot through his ribs.

"You..." He shook his head carefully. "Actually did it, I remember you talking about starting a club someday."

Viper shrugged modestly.

"Took a while but we got there."

Drake instinctively tried to push himself upright and almost immediately another pair of hands rested gently against his bare chest.

"Whoa, tough guy." A woman's warm voice carried a teasing smile. "You're not going anywhere."

Drake turned his head. She smiled down at him. Long, wavy dark brown hair rested over her shoulders. Bright light-blue eyes met his. A beautifully detailed peacock feather tattoo curled along one arm.

She couldn't have been much younger than him. She looked calm. Comfortable. Like she'd done this many times before. Drake relaxed immediately beneath her hands.

"Sorry...I wasn't thinking."

"So I've noticed," she teased.

He couldn't help a faint smile. His attention shifted back to Viper.

"What happened to the Stray Sons?" The question hung in the room. "Where are Hudson and Cullen?"

The smile slowly disappeared from Viper's face. His shoulders sagged ever so slightly.

For several long moments he didn't answer. Finally he looked down at the floor.

"They're dead."

The words landed like a punch. Drake stared silently. His chest tightened. He hadn't known either of them for more than a handful of days all those years ago. Yet those few days had been some of the happiest he'd experienced after leaving Dragonfly Academy.

They had laughed together. Shared motel breakfasts, argued over boxing matches, and played ridiculous pranks on Hudson. Drake had felt like he belonged somewhere and now both of them were gone.

"I'm sorry," Drake said quietly.

Viper nodded once.

"It's a story for another time." His voice made it clear the subject wasn't open for discussion.

Drake respected that. Silence settled over the room. The door opened. A dark-skinned teenage boy stepped inside. His shaggy black hair fell across his forehead and his strangely colored contact lenses instantly reminded Drake of Donovan's demonic red contacts. The resemblance caught him off guard.

"Viper?" The teenager held up a cordless phone. "You have a phone call." His eyes shifted curiously toward Drake. "He's finally awake?"

A grin spread across Viper's face. He stood and wrapped an arm around the teenager's shoulders.

"This," Viper said proudly, "is my stepson, Vance."

Drake looked between them.

"Stepson?" He blinked. "You're married?"

A shadow crossed Viper's expression.

"I was."

The single statement carried far more weight than Drake could understand. Whatever had happened...it still hurt.

Before Drake could ask anything else, Viper lightly patted Vance's shoulder.

"I better take that call." He looked back toward the woman still standing beside Drake's bed. "Just relax. He pointed a finger playfully. "And don't give Estella any problems, okay?"

Estella laughed.

"I think I can handle one stubborn patient."

Drake managed a tired nod.

"I'll behave."

"I'll believe that when I see it," Viper replied with a smirk. He turned and walked toward the door with Vance following close behind. The door clicked softly shut behind them.

The room grew quiet again. Drake stared at the ceiling.

His entire body still ached. His head felt like someone had split it open with an axe. He had no idea how long he had been unconscious.

He didn't know how Viper had found him. He didn't know what had happened after Darius brought that nailed club crashing down onto his skull. Those answers could wait but at least he wasn't looking over his shoulder. He wasn't sleeping with one eye open. He wasn't wondering whether Iron Requiem would burst through the door before morning.

By some miracle, he was alive and somehow, against all odds...he had ended up with the one person from his past he knew he could trust.

Chapter Twenty-Nine

Drake finally began to relax once Estella was satisfied that he had stopped trying to pretend he wasn't injured.

She had fussed over him for several more minutes, making sure he drank another full glass of water before gently fluffing the pillow behind his head. She'd checked the bandage wrapped around his skull, frowned at the ugly bruises spreading across his ribs and shoulders, and warned him more than once that if he didn't stay in bed, she would personally tie him to it.

"I mean it," she had said with one hand on her hip. "You have a fractured skull. You don't get to be stubborn right now."

Drake had managed a tired smirk.

"I've been stubborn my whole life."

She rolled her eyes dramatically before softening again.

"I'll bring you something to eat in a little while. You've been unconscious for days. Your body's going to need it."

He nodded.

"Thanks."

"And stay put."

"I will."

She narrowed her eyes.

"I don't believe you."

"You shouldn't."

That earned him a laugh. She shook her head as she backed toward the door.

"If you need anything, holler. Don't try getting up by yourself."

"I'll be fine."

"You most certainly won't."

With one last disapproving look, she disappeared into the hallway. The room fell quiet once more.

Drake let himself sink into the mattress. The silence felt...Strange. Comfortable. Safe. His eyes drifted closed. Only for a minute. Maybe two. Then his bladder reminded him exactly how much water Estella had insisted he drink.

He sighed. He considered calling for her like she'd instructed. No. It was only the bathroom. He could manage that. He'd survived Dragonfly Academy. Years on the run. Iron Requiem. Surely he could walk twenty feet.

Slowly, he pushed the blankets aside. Every muscle protested. He gritted his teeth and eased himself upright. The room immediately tilted. A pounding ache exploded through his skull. Tiny stars danced across his vision.

"Fuck..." he whispered.

He stayed perfectly still until the dizziness eased enough for him to breathe normally again. Then he swung both legs over the edge of the bed. Only when his feet touched the cool wooden floor did he look down.

Black boxers. White socks. Nothing else.

He frowned.

"Who the hell undressed me?" He muttered the question to himself. He wasn't sure he wanted the answer. Probably Estella. Maybe Jethro. Maybe both. He decided not to think about it. Bracing one hand against the mattress, Drake slowly stood. Pain shot through his body.

His ribs burned. His back screamed. His head felt as though someone were driving railroad spikes straight through it but he remained standing.

"See?" he muttered to himself. "Not so bad..."

The lie barely left his mouth before his knees threatened to buckle. He steadied himself. The bathroom waited at the opposite end of the room but it looked a mile away. One careful step. Another and another. His breathing grew heavier.

The room swayed again. He reached for one of the nearby bedposts, missed, and his legs suddenly gave out.

"Oh, shit—" He toppled sideways. Instead of hitting the floor, he landed squarely on another bed. Someone was already sleeping there.

"Oof!"

The man beneath him jerked awake immediately.

"What in the hell...?"

Strong hands shoved Drake sideways. Drake rolled awkwardly off the mattress before catching himself in a sitting position on the floor. He immediately grabbed his pounding head. Everything spun. The other man sat upright rubbing his eyes.

"What the..."

Then they both froze. Recognition flashed across both faces. Drake stared.

"You have got to be kidding me..."

The man blinked once.

"Donovan?"

"Well..." He shrugged. "Surprise?"

Drake stared another second as Donovan brushed his long silver dyed hair back over his shoulder before stretching with a groan.

"I was hoping you'd wake up under slightly less... dramatic circumstances."

Drake shook his head slowly and immediately regretted it.

"How in hell..." He squinted at Donovan. "Did you know I'd be here?"

"I didn't." Donovan shrugged again. "I joined Venom Bite a few years ago."

That caught Drake completely off guard.

"You did?"

"Yeah and I had no idea Viper even knew you." Donovan leaned back against the headboard. "When we rolled up and found those assholes beating the hell out of you..." He nodded toward Drake. "Viper recognized you first and he made sure we put an end to it immediately."

Drake frowned.

"You went up against Iron Requiem?" There was genuine disbelief in his voice.

Donovan chuckled quietly.

"I helped but honestly..." He smiled faintly. "It was mostly Viper and Lazarus, they're the ones who convinced Iron Requiem to back off."

"Lazarus?"

"Our vice president." Donovan folded his arms. "Trust me, you don't want to be on his bad side."

Drake nodded thoughtfully.

"And Jethro?"

"He's sort of a medic or was gonna be, he was studying to become one but didn't quite finish." Donovan explained. "But he's patched up enough bikers over the years that everyone trusts him, he was the first one working on your head."

Drake let out a slow breath.

"Well..." A tired smile tugged at one corner of his mout. "Damn, I guess I owe you a thank you."

Donovan looked almost offended.

"We're dragon brothers, Drake." His voice grew more serious. "You might not like me and we might never be friends but we survived the same hell and if our positions had been reversed..." He looked Drake directly in the eyes. "I know you'd have done the same for me."

Drake couldn't argue with that. After everything between them...Despite Ambrosia. Despite Helena. Despite all the years of mistrust...He would have helped.

He nodded once.

"Yeah, I would have."

Silence settled between them for a few moments. Then Drake asked quietly,

"Where's Ambrosia?"

Donovan's expression changed instantly. His shoulders stiffened and he looked away.

"We're not together anymore."

Nothing else. Just those four words. Drake watched him carefully. Drake knew that Donovan wasn't being completely honest and he wanted to ask what had happened. Whether she was safe. He opened his mouth but then remembered why he'd gotten out of bed in the first place.

"Actually..." He winced. "I really need the bathroom."

He planted one hand against the mattress and pushed himself upright. The room immediately spun. Dark spots flooded his vision. His knees buckled.

Before he could fall again, Donovan was already on his feet.

"Easy." He caught Drake by the arm. "I've got you."

Drake hesitated only a second before accepting the support. Together they started slowly toward the bathroom. Each careful step sent another wave of pain through Drake's battered body. Even leaning on Donovan, walking felt like climbing a mountain and he couldn't help thinking how strange life was.

Years ago, Donovan had been the one person from Dragonfly Academy he trusted least.

Now...he was the one keeping Drake on his feet.

Chapter Thirty

Drake had not expected recovery to take as long as it had.

The first few weeks after the attack by Iron Requiem had been a blur of headaches, dizziness, and long stretches of sleep. Jethro had checked on him constantly, shining lights in his eyes, changing bandages, and reminding everyone that a fractured skull wasn't something a man simply walked away from because he was stubborn enough.

Drake had tried anyway.

More than once Estella had caught him attempting to carry boxes, help clean the clubhouse, or work on his Harley before his balance betrayed him. Every single time she had marched him right back to bed with a lecture that reminded him a little too much of a mother fussing over her son.

Now, nearly three months after Venom Bite had pulled him away from what should have been his death at the hands of Darius Crowe, life finally felt...steady.

He still occupied one of the beds in the large bunkroom at the clubhouse. The room smelled faintly of cigarette smoke, leather, laundry detergent, and coffee. Boots sat beneath nearly every bed, duffel bags were tucked against the walls, and someone's music drifted faintly from another room.

Earlier that afternoon, Jethro had finished another examination.

The former medical student had made Drake follow his finger with his eyes, checked his pupils one last time, pressed carefully around the old fracture, and finally leaned back with a satisfied nod.

"Well," Jethro had said, pulling off a pair of gloves, "I officially hate admitting when you're right."

Drake smirked.

"So that's it?"

"You're cleared."

Drake let out a slow breath.

"Finally."

Jethro pointed a finger at him.

"That doesn't mean you're invincible."

"I know."

"No, you don't."

Drake laughed quietly. Jethro continued.

"The fracture has healed well. Your ribs are good, everything has closed up exactly how I hoped it would." He folded his arms. "But..."

"There it is," Drake muttered.

"But," Jethro repeated, "head injuries can be unpredictable. If you start getting severe headaches, blurred vision, confusion, vomiting, blackouts, you tell me immediately."

"I will."

"And don't go looking for fights."

Drake raised an eyebrow.

"You've met me."

"Exactly why I'm saying it."

Drake couldn't help laughing.

"I'll try."

Jethro snorted.

"I'll believe that when I see it."

That evening the clubhouse had settled into its usual rhythm. Several members played pool. Someone argued over a card game near the bar. Music played from an old jukebox tucked into the corner.

The smell of burgers drifted in from the kitchen while laughter echoed through the building. Drake stood near the bar nursing a bottle of beer. Sometimes a sharp pain would flash behind his eyes without warning, but compared to where he'd been months earlier, he felt like a different man.

A familiar voice interrupted his thoughts.

"So you're all good now then?"

Drake looked over.

Viper leaned casually against the bar with a beer in one hand. His orange-streaked hair caught the light, and despite everything life had thrown at him over the years, he somehow still managed to grin like the world hadn't beaten him down.

Drake shrugged.

"Guess so." He rubbed the back of his neck. "Though I still get headaches now and then."

Viper nodded.

"Jethro said that might happen for a while."

"He also threatened to glue me to the bed if I start another fight."

Viper laughed.

"Sounds like him."

There was a comfortable silence between them. It felt different than the awkward conversations they'd shared years earlier when the Stray Sons consisted of only Viper, Hudson, and Cullen.

Back then they'd barely known each other. Now Drake trusted him with his life. Viper took another drink before speaking again.

"Well, good."

Drake glanced over.

"Good?"

"Yeah." Viper set his bottle down. "Because you have to go through initiation."

Drake blinked.

"Excuse me?"

Viper looked genuinely confused by his reaction.

"What?"

"I've been living here for three months."

"Yep." Viper nodded.

"You guys patched me up."

"Yep."

"I've eaten your food."

"Yep." Viper continued to nod.

"I've watched Vance cheat at cards."

"I heard that!" Vance yelled from across the room.

"You did cheat!" Drake called back.

"I was winning!"

"You hid three aces in your sleeve."

Vance looked offended.

"I was strategically storing them."

The room erupted into laughter. Viper shook his head.

"Anyway..." He looked back at Drake. "Initiation."

Drake folded his arms.

"I thought I was already in."

"As far as I'm concerned, you are." Viper leaned one shoulder against the bar. "But the others weren't around back when we met."

Drake nodded slowly.

"They don't know about the Stray Sons."

"They just don't know you." Viper said.

"They don't know you trusted me before Venom Bite even existed."

"No, they just know you're some big bald guy we rescued from Iron Requiem."

Drake sighed.

"So then..." he asked. "What do I have to do?" A suspicious look crossed his face. "You're not gonna have me do something ridiculous like moving railroad ties are you?"

For a second Viper simply stared. Then he burst into laughter. He laughed so hard he nearly spilled his beer.

Drake waited patiently. Finally Viper caught his breath.

"Oh...no." He wiped a tear from his eye. "We like to brawl."

Drake raised an eyebrow.

"That's...slightly reassuring."

Viper grinned.

"It's tradition, usually Lazarus handles challengers."

Across the room Lazarus looked up from his conversation.

"I heard my name."

"You'll hear it again," Viper called and Lazarus rolled his eyes. "Sometimes Donovan does it," Viper continued. "But he already refused."

Drake looked surprised.

"He refused?"

Viper nodded.

"Said he wasn't going up against you."

A grin slowly spread across Drake's face.

"Smart man."

Viper laughed.

"He said he's been on the receiving end when people underestimate you."

"I've mellowed."

Lazarus snorted loudly.

"No, you haven't."

The room chuckled again. Viper continued.

"I honestly don't think Lazarus will beat you."

Lazarus pointed toward himself.

"Hey!" He exclaimed in an offended tone.

"You're strong," Viper said. "But Drake's built like somebody carved him out of a mountain."

Drake smirked.

"I'll take that as a compliment."

"It is." Viper shrugged. "And besides...it's mostly for show."

Drake looked at him.

"What do you mean?"

"It's not some death match." Viper waved dismissively. "It's more like two stubborn idiots wrestling until one gives up."

"So...no knives."

"No."

"No bats with nails."

"Definitely not."

"No railroad ties."

Viper laughed again.

"No railroad ties."

Drake let out a relieved breath.

"Well...I suppose I can handle that."

"You'll probably enjoy it." Viper said.

"Maybe."

Viper picked up his beer again.

"So whenever you're ready, no rush, I don't want that bald head of yours breaking again."

Drake chuckled.

"Sure thing..." He looked thoughtfully at Viper's bright orange streaks. "Flamethrower."

Viper froze.

"What?"

"Your hair, the bright orange streaks, they look like fire."

Viper groaned dramatically.

"Oh, absolutely not."

"What?"

"They call me Snake around here because of my name and because of my father...he went by Python when he was president of this MC."

Drake nodded thoughtfully.

"Still think Flamethrower fits."

Lazarus laughed loud enough for the room to hear.

"I'm calling him that now."

"You are not," Viper shot back.

"Too late," Donovan added from a nearby table with a grin. Several members immediately started chanting.

"Flame."

"Thrower."

"Flame."

"Thrower."

Viper buried his face in one hand.

"I hate all of you."

The clubhouse filled with laughter. Even Drake laughed harder than he had in years. It felt...good. Normal. Something he'd almost forgotten existed.

Eventually the laughter died down.

Viper smiled.

"Seriously though, get some rest and when you're ready, we'll do the initiation." He paused. "Oh and one more thing."

Drake looked up.

"There's already a patched vest waiting for you."

Drake stared at him.

"What?"

"It's hanging in my office, has been for weeks, I was just waiting for Jethro to clear you."

For a long moment Drake couldn't find any words. He had spent so many years drifting from one highway to another. Always alone. Always temporary. Never belonging anywhere. Now someone had already prepared a place for him before he'd even earned it.

Viper clapped him on the shoulder.

"We knew you weren't leaving." Then he walked away toward the pool tables.

Drake remained standing by the bar, staring after him. His throat tightened unexpectedly. He looked around the noisy clubhouse.

Men arguing over pool. Someone laughing in the kitchen. Vance trying to convince everyone he hadn't cheated. Lazarus already calling Viper "Flamethrower" just to annoy him.

Drake took a deep breath and exhaled as he realized that wasn't wondering where he'd sleep tomorrow. He wasn't wondering where the next road would take him. He wasn't wondering who might be chasing him and he quietly smiled to himself.

He finally knew.

He was home.

The End?

End of Book

We truly appreciate you taking the time to read Dust, Scars, And A Place To Land. We hope you enjoyed the journey through Drake's past and that you will be along for the ride when his story continues.

If this story captivated you, we would be incredibly grateful if you could take a moment to rate and review it. Your feedback not only helps other readers discover the book, but it also means the world to us as writers.

Thank you for your support, and we hope to share more stories with you soon!

— Mindy M. Mather & Maranda Florer

Other Books In This Series

Book 1: Roche Pride

Book 2: Sons of the Asphalt

Book 3: Blood & Betrayal

Book 4: The Price of Legacy

Related Books

Pride of the Lion (Prequel to Roche Pride)

Loyalty is a Lie

Ace of Diamonds (Coincides with Legacy is a Lie)

Dust, Scars, And A Place To Land (This Book)

Made in the USA
Monee, IL
12 November 2026

5ed1a746-afb8-427c-94e5-c2cb851ab9e4R01